KT-568-271

SlimmingWorld

Food Optimising

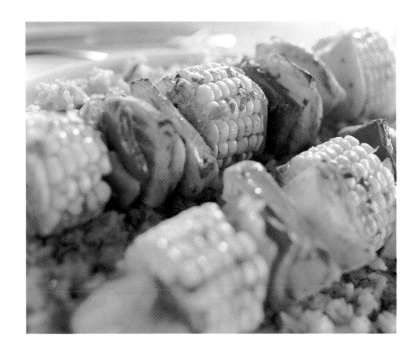

Slimming World

Food Optimising

The satisfying way to

lose weight and feel great with

over 120 delicious recipes

EBURY PRESS

Published in 2000 by Ebury Press, an imprint of Ebury Publishing

A Random House Group company

Text © Slimming World 2000
Food photography © Random House Group Ltd/Daniel Pangbourne 2000
Other photography, see acknowledgements on page 224

The Random House Group Limited Reg. No. 954009

Addresses for companies within the Random House Group can be found at penguinrandomhouse.com

A CIP catalogue record for this book is available from the British Library.

FOR SLIMMING WORLD
Editorial direction Margaret Miles-Bramwell
Contributing editor Claire Crowther
Nutritionist Jacqui Lavin MMedSci. PhD RNutr.
Food co-ordination Allison Brentnall
Menu developer Emma Naylor
Recipe development Kathryn Hawkins
Food photography advisor Diane Brown

FOR EBURY PRESS
Editor Emma Callery
Designer Alison Shackleton
Stylist Tessa Evelegh
Food economist Val Barrett
Picture research Claire Taylor

ISBN 9780091872540

Penguin Random House is committed to a sustainable future for our business,
our readers and our planet. This book is made from Forest Stewardship
Council® certified paper.

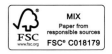

Printed and bound in China by C&C Offset Printing Co., Ltd

To buy books by your favourite authors and register for offers visit www.penguin.co.uk

Contents

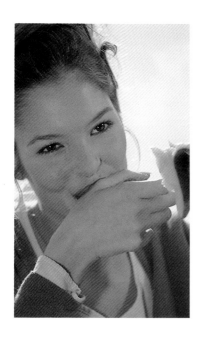

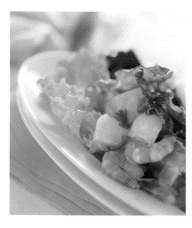

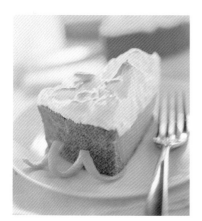

foreword

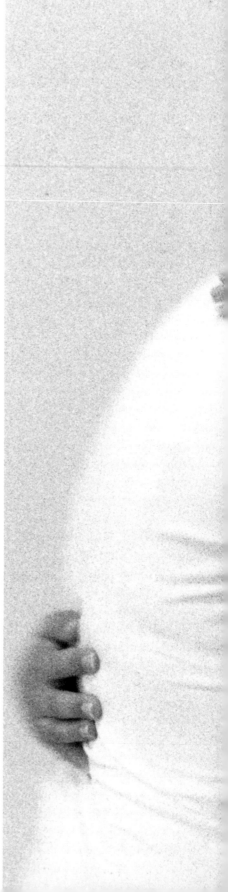

Dear Reader,

I haven't met you, yet I want to thank you personally for two things: for deciding this book can help you slim effectively and for taking a moment or two with me.

I believe that this book will be of lifelong value to you. Actually, you are enormously valuable to me. Every day of my life for the past forty years, I have woken up and begun a day's conversation with you – you, the everyday slimmer, the woman or man in the street who, like me, lives a life that's pushed towards weight and longs for a body that's never put on an extra ounce. When I was young, it was you who gave me hope, for I realised I wasn't alone in my struggle. Since 1969 my personal life goal has been to forge a path forward for anybody caught up in the diet trap and the misery of excess weight.

There isn't a slimming dilemma that I haven't experienced. There isn't a day I don't wish for a magic bullet because I'm an everyday slimmer, because I've struggled with overweight, because I feel nobody should go through such struggles alone. So I'm delighted to share with you this incredible system of Food Optimising which I, as a food lover, know to be the kindest, most effective weight loss system possible. Hundreds of thousands of men and women have used it, lost weight and live by its principles.

I'm pleased – but not surprised – to say that nutritionists agree with our findings at Slimming World. They have ensured our methods are in line with current nutritional thinking. But it's not just a matter of nutrition, important though that is. Losing weight successfully is about motivation, enjoyment and letting ourselves off all the hooks we slimmers get stuck on.

I am delighted to share Food Optimising with you in book form as we at Slimming World have been sharing it, week in, week out, for so many years. Find out why Food Optimising is the nearest thing to a magic wand you'll every need. Discover the joy of weight loss without hunger. Experience the thrill of those inches melting away. Enjoy the liberation that your new self-confidence brings. Become, at last and for ever, the person you really want to be.

Use this book to the full and we promise the only thing that will grow larger will be your self-esteem.

There's really only one thing you need to remember – you can do it.

Warmest wishes

Margaret Miles-Bramwell

FOUNDER OF SLIMMING WORLD

Photograph by Lord Lichfield

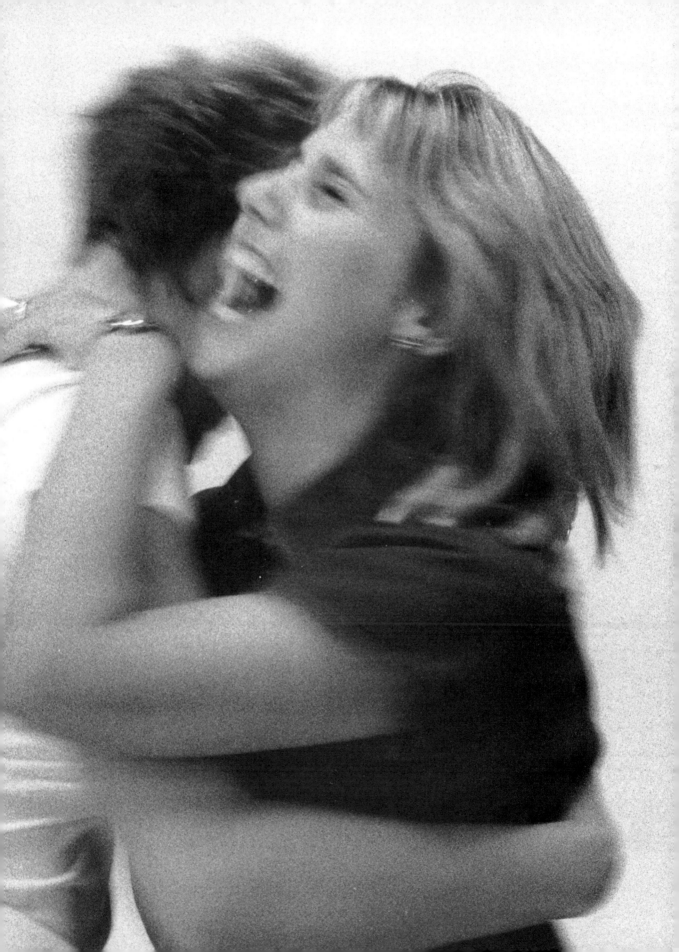

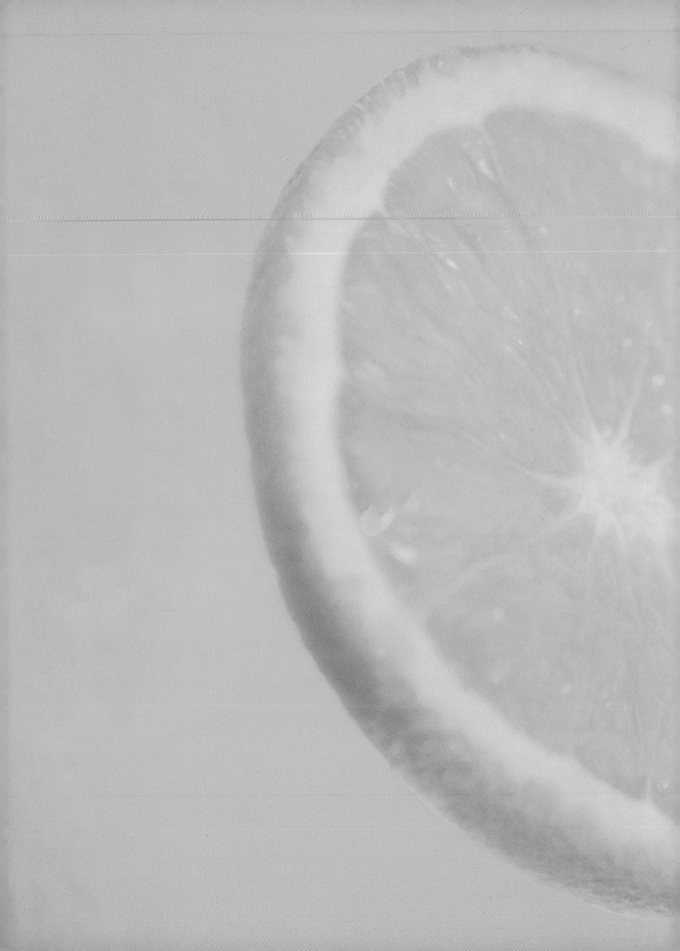

chapter 1

the benefits of food optimising

1 the benefits of food optimising

Would you like to:
- *Eat to satisfy your appetite?*
- *Eat in the way slim people do?*
- *Choose foods you personally enjoy each day?*
- *Know you are eating in the healthiest way known to nutritionists?*

If you answer yes to these questions then Food Optimising is a way of losing weight that will work for you. It is designed to give you:
- *Satisfaction, so you never allow yourself to go hungry again.*
- *Freedom and relaxation around food just as slim people have.*
- *Personal preference in what you can eat freely within the larger food groups, such as pasta, potato or meat.*
- *Your choice, every single day, of your favourite treats.*

Food Optimising goes further than freedom, satisfaction and personal preference. It is founded on very sophisticated concepts about how and why we overeat. This is the heart of Food Optimising. When you find yourself wondering why a certain food is free when other diets tell you to cut it down, you will have hit on Food Optimising in action. This way of losing weight has forty years of development behind it. Slimming World knows as much as there is to know about the way overeating, dieting and healthy eating interact in practice. We know just how you will feel when you start eating instead of starving to lose weight. We know how you need to eat to succeed and also how you will want to eat to stay slim long term. All these factors are built into our Food Optimising programme.

Food Optimising is the most slimmer-friendly eating system there is

Food Optimising is only available at Slimming World. Its unique and sophisticated method was devised and developed at Slimming World headquarters in Derbyshire and continues to be practised by thousands – hundreds of thousands – of slimmers of all ages at Slimming World groups that are held weekly right across Britain.

Slimming World was begun back in 1969 and its basic principles have never changed, although Food Optimising has been developed in accordance with the changing guidelines of orthodox nutrition. In fact, you can be assured that if you decide to try Food Optimising, you will be eating in the way that is thought to be the healthiest for people wanting to lose weight today.

Heap that plate and dump the pain-gain legacy

In the Seventies and Eighties, slimming was thought to be a matter of painful food restriction – the lower the calorie intake, the better was the prevailing philosophy. Sadly, this legacy of pain-gain slimming has held on and we know from experience just how many people really deeply believe that they have to go hungry and feel deprived to lose weight.

We have always known that, if you have a weight problem, what you want is lots of gorgeous food – and having far too little of it is not a course of action that could possibly last long. Your body would crave the comfort of a really satisfying meal and your mind would be tormented by the food you were being denied.

That's not the way to get slim and stay slim. Restricting intake too much results in the loss of more lean tissue (such as muscle) from our bodies as well as body fat. Loss of lean tissue has unfavourable effects on our metabolic rate: the more we lose, the more our metabolic rate will fall. This is why experts recommend gradual weight loss on a sensible calorie intake – and not severely calorie-restricted (crash) diets.

Furthermore, dieting in this way makes it a lot harder to get all your vital nutrients. At Slimming World, the normal desire for heaped platefuls is treated with respect and, indeed, the fact that you can learn how to heap up your plate freely on a regular basis while actually losing weight is one factor that has produced devoted Food Optimisers.

And we really mean Free. You eat as much as you like, when you like, as often as you like when you eat Free Foods (see box on pages 42-3). There is absolutely no need to weigh or measure them – you will lose weight if you satisfy your appetite with our Free Foods.

Manage those calories and bin that calorie-counter

Do you hate the very word calorie? Most of us have had a run-in with calorie counting at some point during our search for a slimmer shape. In fact, calorie counting is possibly the most hated way to lose weight. Yet all experts agree that you have to lower your calorie intake in order to lose weight. But how can you achieve this and not run out of things to eat by mid-afternoon?

Foods are used to gain maximum benefit from these processes

> ### What Food Optimising means
>
> ✓ The Food Optimising plan is divided into Green days and Original days.
>
> ✓ Simply decide whether you want to have a Green or Original day and stick to that choice all day.
>
> ✓ You can make every day a Green day, or have a mixture of Green and Original days.
>
> ✓ Pick your recipes according to which day you choose (see menus on pages 34-41 and recipe charts on pages 218-211).
>
> ✓ Pile you plate with Free Foods, eating as much of these as you want (see pages 42-3).
>
> ✓ Choose Speed Foods to give your weight loss an even bigger boost (see pages 42-3).
>
> ✓ Enjoy Syns: through Food Optimising you are allowed a daily quota of treats (see pages 42-3).

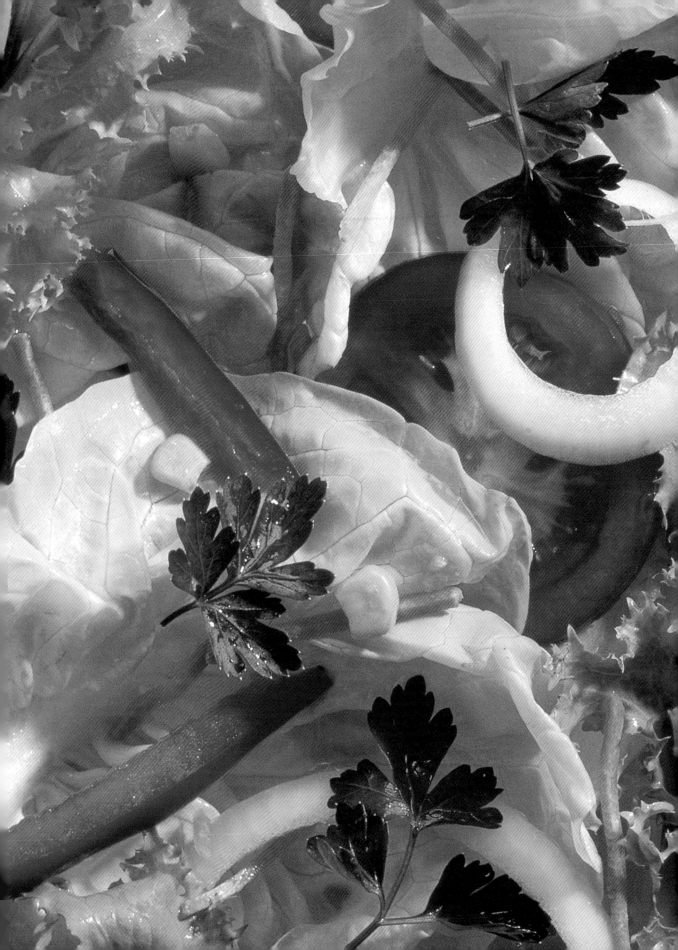

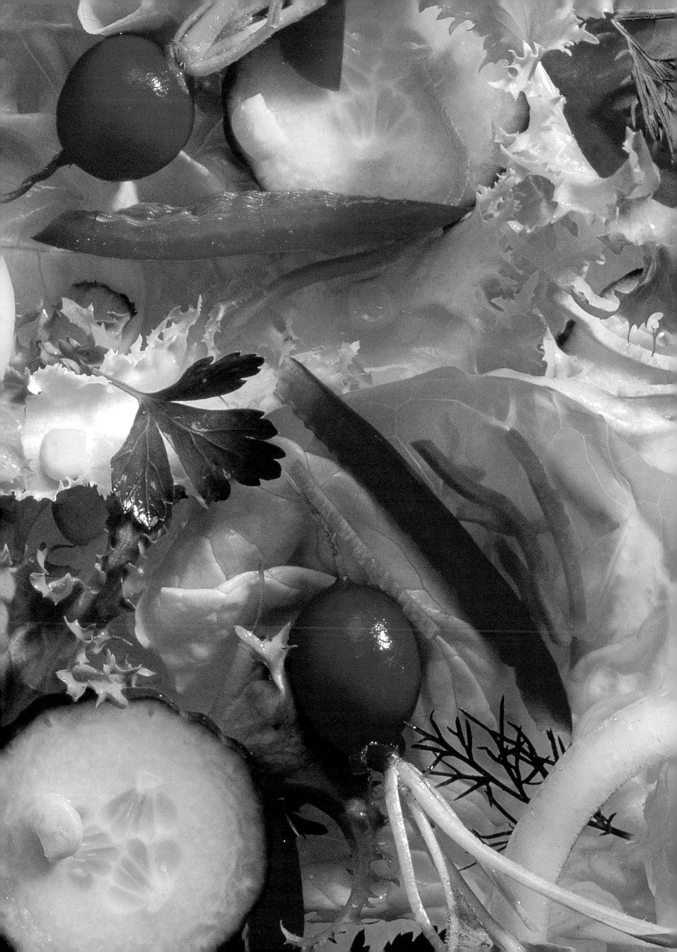

Yes, you can eat fewer calories while filling up. You can carry on eating even till late at night. Recent research indicates that late-night eating is no more fattening than taking in those same calories earlier in the day. Food Optimising works because it helps you learn how to satisfy your appetite by making healthy food choices, which naturally limit your calorie intake. Scientific research has shown that there are many signals that arise as we eat, digest and absorb food, which work together to suppress our appetite. These signals stop us eating a meal when our body doesn't need any more (that's called satiation) and prevent us from eating again until our body requires more energy (known as satiety). Food Optimising incorporates the latest scientific understanding of how foods trigger the signals that regulate our appetite.

Because your appetite is satisfied, you will find yourself comfortably limiting your calorie intake – without counting a single calorie. Our menus in this book are all the proof you'll need. Just use them every day and watch your weight drop.

Choose your food

The joy of Food Optimising is that you choose the foods you really like and some of those choices you will eat without any other restriction than your appetite. Like to nibble on chicken? Go for it. Love more than a couple of potatoes? No problem. Then you can add some Healthy Extras, and on top of that, let's not forget those treats.

In this way, you'll come to understand that you can have as varied a plateful as a slim person, that you can

Feel full – eat – enjoy getting slim – love staying slim

'I'd never had that kind of weight loss without starving'

Melanie Valenti weighed 23 stones when she joined Slimming World in 1996 and began Food Optimising. 'I'd tried various diets but I didn't understand which foods were fattening so I'd have a salad with a huge chunk of cheese or crispbreads plastered with butter. For each stone I lost, I put on two more once the diet ended.
I instantly felt at home with Food Optimising –

unlimited foods, so I never had to go hungry. In my first week I lost 9 pounds and I was hooked. I knew some of that loss was water but I soon settled into an average of two pounds loss a week and now I weigh 10st 5lbs. I'd never before had that kind of weight loss without starving myself. I couldn't believe I could eat so much and still lose weight.'

Melanie, who is 5ft 5in, lost 13 stones with Food Optimising.

choose smaller portions of some foods knowing thatreally super filling and great-tasting food is on offer all day long – and you will learn how to handle food in this way forever.

That's the good part – Food Optimising is designed to work forever. It's long-term healthy eating, it's your eating lifestyle for the twenty-first century, and not just when you are following menus made for you. Check the lists and explore the possibilities of personal preference.

Food Optimising is based on dividing foods into groups:
- Foods that fill you so well, you can eat as much as you like of them.
- Foods that typically all diets ban.
- Foods that speed your weight loss.
- Foods that boost vitamins and minerals, calcium and fibre.

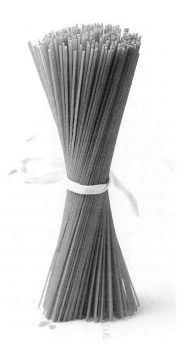

All you have to do is choose what you'd like to eat from these enormous lists, which include absolutely everything! So you just can't miss out! Members of Slimming World groups quickly learn how to handle the lists to make whatever meals they want every day – to fit in with their personal preferences, their family's needs and tastes, whether they're having a quick lunch, a TV dinner or entertaining.

In Chapter Three, we have constructed menus from our most popular dishes and each one is built on the unique Food Optimising principles and lists. So that you can try the freedom of Food Optimising, we have also included a list of Free Foods and a list of treats for you to swap within. Remember, if you become a Slimming World member, your choices will be much wider than this and you will be able to make up all your own menus every day if you wish.

As you work with these groups of foods to make up your own preferred daily menus, you will learn exactly which foods work to satisfy your hunger and your taste buds while they change that steady weight gain into an amazing weight loss.

Prove to yourself the benefits of Food Optimising – that slimming doesn't have to be boring salad after salad, day in, day out. This book provides great ready-made menus (see pages 34-41) and recipes together with a basic set of foods to practise with.

Because Food Optimising recipes are based on the very best principles of nutrition, they can be used even if you don't want to lose weight. Your family will enjoy them too. Eating in this way helps you to keep a stable weight through life. Most of us worry that we will put on weight as we get older – but that's no longer inevitable. In fact, with Food Optimising, you're in the driving seat – for good!

'My plate is now twice as full as it used to be'

Gail Graver, who lost 10st 8lbs by Food Optimising, had tried calorie counting and even slimming pills. Nothing worked. She was enduring constant discomfort and heartburn and yet, as she says, 'I'd never eaten huge quantities – I just ate unhealthily. My plate now is twice as full as it used to be and I enjoy my food more than I used to. I enjoy the variety of Food Optimising.'

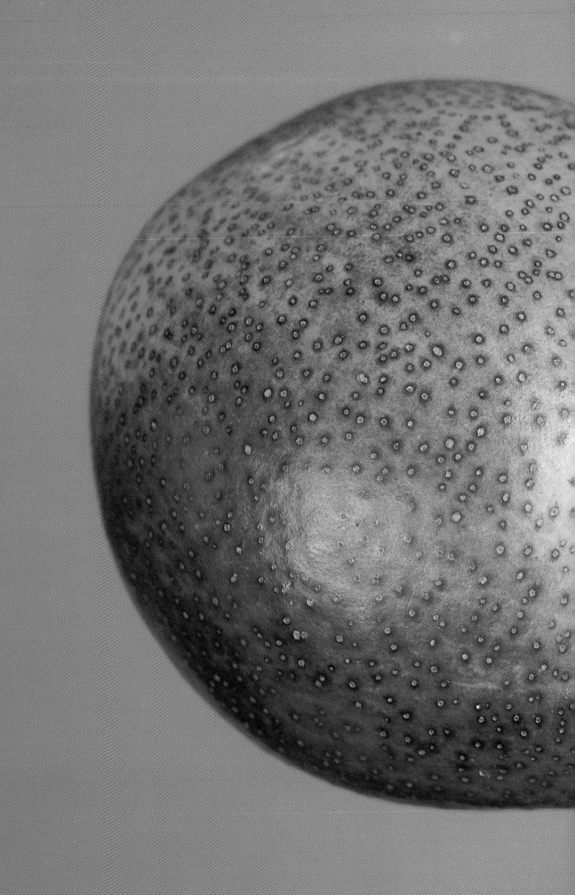

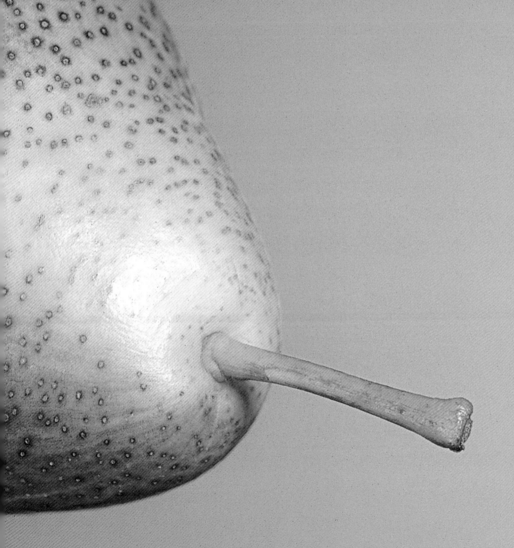

chapter 2

the secrets of food optimising

2 The secrets of Food Optimising

Food Optimising is what you will be doing as you eat these recipes, follow the menus and watch your weight go down. Soon it will become a habit, easy and comfortable, every day and for life. There is no need to know in-depth nutrition theory or calculate food values – that has all been done for you. If you practise Food Optimising, you will come instinctively to know how to adjust your balance of foods to stay slim.

If you prefer, you can go straight to the menus that start on page 34 and start Food Optimising right now. However, if you'd like to know some whys and wherefores, take the time to read this chapter. It could help your commitment to healthy eating.

Filling or fattening?

Why is one plateful fattening and another, with the same quantity of food on it, filling yet slimming? A Food Optimising plateful will be full, but it is what it is filled with that counts. On a Green day it will be full of unlimited potatoes or pasta or rice with loads of whatever vegetables take your fancy plus a measured amount of meat or fish. A similar plateful, but this time of unlimited meat or fish with a measured amount of pasta or potato and heaped again with vegetables, will be a great Original day of Food Optimising.

Food Optimising only stops working when you stop Food Optimising

The comment you're likely to get from non-slimmers around you is, 'Are you sure you're on a diet?' Well, if they mean a weight-reducing diet, then yes, you most certainly are. If they mean a starvation diet, then no you definitely are not! It's the very reason why thousands of satisfied slimmers exclaim, 'You cannot possibly call this a diet!' What you'll find is that you'll feel full quicker and that feeling of fullness lasts hours longer.

So, what's the difference between this and the fattening plateful? It's the fat, the sugar and the non-filling but calorie-laden elements in the food. Fill your plate with potato, vegetables and meat and plenty of concentrated calories (masquerading as sauce) and you'll feel less satisfied for a much shorter time – and add on those inches. When you're feeling hungry again, which will be in a much shorter time, you'll need a snack to keep you going. Snack in between on crisps or chocolate or biscuits and you'll find that not only do they not satisfy your hunger, they create it. And your weight will soar.

When your appetite has disappeared, not through pills or potions, but through eating the Food Optimising way, you'll then find that you will have more than enough Syns (see box on page 11) to count a chocolate bar into your day – if you can squeeze it in! Just see what happens when you heap up your extra large snack box with this version of Chinese pancakes with crispy duck. Try wrapping slices of cooked chicken (instead of the duck), cucumber and onions in a crisp lettuce leaf spread with a little Hoisin sauce, pack some very low-fat natural fromage frais then add some of your favourite fresh fruit as a dessert and watch the weight just fall off. When you are Food Optimising, the difference is not in quantity but in quality.

Food Optimising meals and snacks will not only satisfy you when you eat them, you'll stay full so much longer. You'll never need to feel ravenous mid-morning or late evening ever again. You will, with no pain or suffering, automatically reduce all those calories that were in excess of your body needs. You will lose weight.

When you are Food Optimising, your body will recognise quickly the energy-giving, appetite-soothing carbohydrates and proteins and give your brain a clear message: 'I can stop eating. I don't need any more. I've had enough.' Whereas after a high-fat snack or meal, the absolute opposite is true. 'More, more!' our brains tell us. In fact, high-fat salty snacks are a common 'trigger' food for many people. Just one or two salty crisps, for example, can start a craving, and with no effective appetite satisfaction signalling, our bodies simply don't register that we are piling in the calories and the whole experience leaves us simply wanting more. Our bodies just don't seem to wake up to a delivery of fat – so we just continue to go on eating.

The problem is that fat is energy dense. It has more than twice as many calories per gram as carbohydrates and protein. You eat a lot more calories from fat before you feel full than you do when you eat carbohydrate or protein. So, the amount of fat in your meal can affect the total amount you eat in that same meal.

Low fat – high carbohydrate

Research at Leeds University shows that, when allowed to eat freely, people eat a lot more calories if foods chosen are higher in fat than if their food is higher in carbohydrates. This was confirmed in a longer term study where 13 women were given either a low-fat diet on a medium-fat diet for 11 weeks and vise versa. Energy intake on the low-fat diet resulted in twice the weight loss than that on the medium-fat diet.

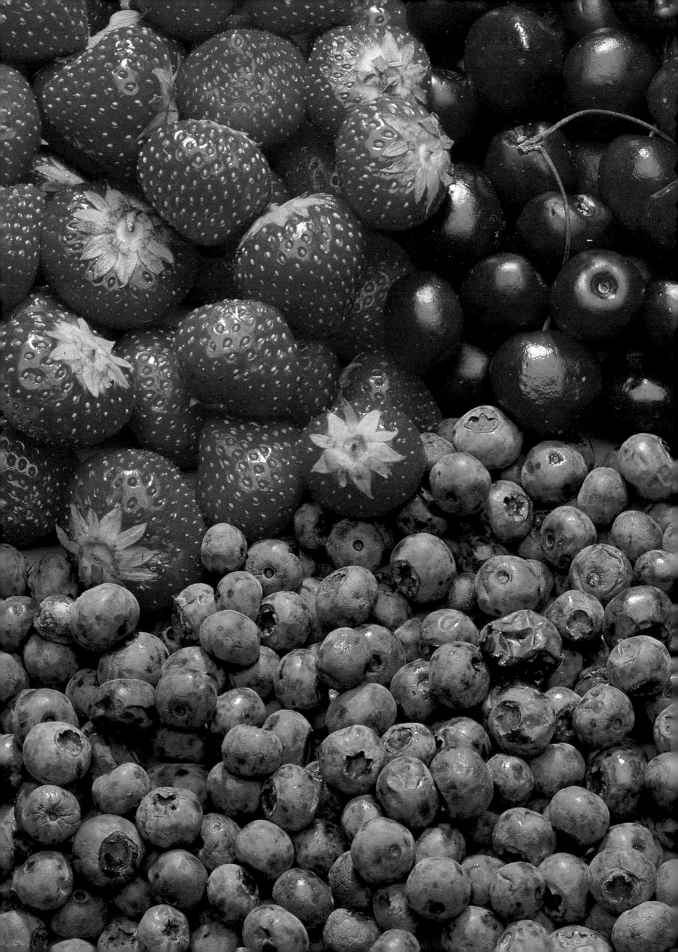

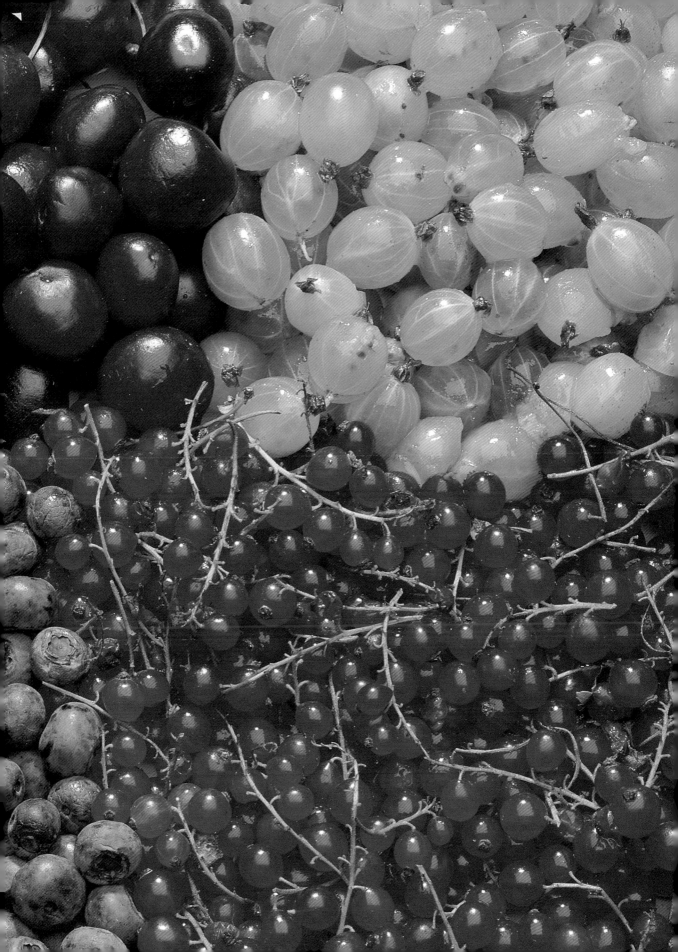

As well as fat not providing the best 'stop eating' messages, high-fat meals may not keep you feeling full for as long as protein and carbohydrate. These foods are not only likely to keep your appetite satisfied for longer, so avoiding those snack cravings, but also the researchers at Leeds University found the subjects of the several experiments ate less at the next meal if they had substituted carbohydrate foods for fat.

Protein power

Protein is satiating (it fills you effectively as you eat) and helps you feel full for longer, just as do carbohydrates. So basing your meals around protein rich foods will help you not to overeat. The British Nutrition Foundation's Task Force Report on Obesity (1999) says: 'Studies have generally shown that protein is the most satiating of the macronutrients followed closely by carbohydrate and then, trailing well behind, fat.'

Foods that contain plenty of protein

Meat – beef, pork, lamb	Tofu
Fish – white and oily	Eggs
Beans, peas and lentils	Nuts
Offal – liver and kidney	Cheese
Quorn	

Clever with carbohydrates

Because complex carbohydrates such as pasta and potatoes are much bulkier than refined carbohydrates like sugar, they can help you feel fuller. They usually contain plenty of fibre, and this adds bulk and helps suppress our appetite. Fibre slows both the digestion and absorption of food and gives us a more gradual release of sugar into the bloodstream as the carbohydrate you've eaten breaks down – and this helps suppress appetite for longer.

The rate at which sugars rise in your blood, and the length of time they are raised after eating carbohydrate-rich foods is called the glycaemic index (GI). A high GI is thought to be less useful in controlling appetite than a low GI. Some diets are based on the glycaemic index. A low, long drawn out GI after eating carbohydrate-rich foods is associated with feelings of satisfaction. For example, apples have a lower GI than apple purée or apple juice and they have been shown to suppress your appetite more effectively. So you get far more benefit from eating fruits in their original form and that's why Food Optimising encourages you to eat whole fruits rather than juices.

Food Optimising also encourages you to choose foods high in complex carbohydrates and fibre, which give you a more gradual and

---

TIPS
• *Today, most fresh meat is lean.*
• *Avoid meat pies and pasties, which have lots of added fat.*
• *Grill instead of fry.*
• *Steam fish.*
• *Non-meat proteins, such as quorn, tofu and beans are often low in fat. Give them a go.*

TIP
Don't be frightened of snacks. If you feel hungry between meals, take a minute or so to assess whether you're reacting to boredom or a trigger such as the clock striking twelve! If you remain hungry, choose a snack from the Free Foods list on page 42 and enjoy it. Eating a meal or snack that is low in fat and based on a complex carbohydrate food whenever you need it will not stop you losing weight. It's what you eat, not how often or when, that counts.

sustained rise in your blood sugar levels. There are several ways it maximises the role of GI in your search for satisfying, slimming meals. It encourages you to eat foods of a less processed kind such as apples rather than juice. It encourages you to choose fibre-rich foods by using an F/FF symbols to guide your choice. And it helps you avoid quick fixes of sugary foods, which cause your blood sugar levels to rise quickly, giving you a high GI. This may satisfy you initially but will be followed by a rapid drop, leaving you begging for more again.

All of these studies of our digestive processes show that we don't necessarily eat more food to gain weight – but we do eat more calories through our choice of food. Food Optimising helps you choose the foods that will satisfy you enough to lose weight while enjoying eating as much as you want.

Foods that contain plenty of carbohydrates

Pasta	Cereals and oats
Noodles	Bread
Rice	Beans, peas and lentils
Potatoes and sweet potatoes	Grains, e.g. millet and couscous
Yams	

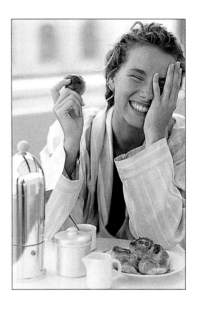

Food Optimising with your appetite

• Learn to recognise false appetite. Ask yourself do I really want to eat or am I hungry because someone else is eating/I am bored/I always eat when the television is on/I always eat at seven o'clock?

• Give yourself a chance to recognise the signs of being really full – take time to eat, chew thoroughly.

• If you're not sure how hungry you are, and you have eaten a meal recently, do something else for 10 minutes then check your appetite – if it's still there, eat.

• Be aware of what foods you personally enjoy that fill you quickly and what foods keep you full for longest. Make a list of your favourites and try to keep that list growing.

The Food Optimising way, you stay in control, you enjoy life, and you continue to lose weight.

• Try to eat foods that need chewing as this helps stimulate the physiology of your appetite to work.

• Although you are following menus in this book, you have a lot of leeway to have more or less of the Free Foods. Use your appetite to guide you and don't be afraid to experiment with it.

• Top carbohydrate fillers are beans, lentils, wholemeal pasta and spaghetti and brown rice. Potatoes boiled in their skins are better than mashed.

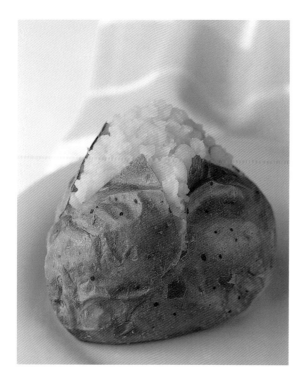

• Eat whole fruits rather than drinking fruit juices as your daily choice of fruit.

Why are some foods listed as Speed Foods?

Losing weight too fast is counterproductive. But lose steadily and you are far more likely to keep your weight off. Using Food Optimising to its full capacity will probably mean you lose between 500g and 1kg/1 and 2lb a week. The first week could see your weight drop by as much as 3 to 4.5kg/7 to 10lb and although much of this will be fluid, it's a great start and will stabilise to a steady loss of fat.

Never, never crash diet. It isn't possible when you're Food Optimising. Slimming World always gives you full responsibility for deciding how much you eat, so we can only advise that eating too little is unhealthy and doesn't work long term.

However, you may want to step up your weight loss at some point – perhaps it has slowed down and you don't know why. So, we have built in Speed choices and Super Speed choices. On the lists given on pages 42-3, you will find some of these marked S and SS. In this book we have included a selection of Speed Foods taken from the full listings (for further information see page 221). The wonderful thing about these Speed Foods is that they contain fewer calories compared to other foods of their type. Fill up on these and you will give your weight loss a boost.

Syn or sanity?

Syns are unique to Slimming World, and they're what makes Food Optimising such an effective weight plan. Syn is short for synergy – the word that describes what happens when the combined effect of individual elements is more powerful than they would be on their own. There's nothing 'sinful' about Syns – far from it. They're a safety net that takes the guilt out of enjoying a glass of wine, a chocolate bar or a packet of crisps, and having Syns ensures you needn't miss out on little extras, like mayo in your sandwich or pepper sauce on your steak. They also ensure that Food Optimising is sustainable in the long term, because no one has to deprive themselves of their favourite treats.

Syns are possibly the most realistic attempt ever by a slimming organisation to stand shoulder to shoulder with its customers. Eating too much, eating the 'wrong' foods, breaking a diet in any one of a thousand ways were activities that were universal and universally despised by non-slimmers. Not only non-slimmers – even other weight-loss organisations

---

Food Optimising with Speed Foods

✓ *Choose S or SS foods from the lists on pages 42-3.*

✓ *Vary the Speed Foods you choose from day to day.*

✓ *Use Speed Foods as snacks or add them to other meals in as large quantities as you like.*

and so-called 'experts' can still have so little understanding of the problem of weight that they use humiliation and punishment as supposed inducements to slim successfully. Not surprisingly, these terrorist tactics are bound to fail, and it is slimmers who are left carrying the burden and guilt of failure.

Countless slimmers have believed their inability to stick to a diet was entirely their fault. This approach is damaging to self-esteem and therefore to weight loss. Food Optimising takes this serious situation and lightens it – in more ways than one.

Syns takes the guilt right out of eating. They're also something you choose to have whenever you want – and as long as you're aware of how many Syns you are consuming and keep them within your allocation you'll carry on losing weight. Keeping a daily log of your Syn count is an excellent way to stay aware – we slimmers have an ability to develop what some cynics might term 'selective amnesia'! And the allocation of Syns? Just like your target weight, it's your decision. Some days you'll be happy on as few as five, other days you'll need a more generous amount, maybe even 25 or 30. As long as you keep counting and don't forget about them altogether, you and your weight loss will be safe.

Unlike calorie counting, you only count Syns, those foods that are too high in fats, or sugars, or simply don't have the filling power for the amount of calories they dispense. And unlike calorie counting, where you never subconsciously learn which foods are the best for you, you will soon come to appreciate which foods have those hidden and unnecessary calories that are surplus to requirements and so end up as unwanted layers of fat on your body.

Cutting down on the volume of food you eat, which is what happens when you count calories, has been shown time and time again to be the slimmer's worst enemy and the biggest single reason for failure. Counting calories creates a constant and unnatural focus on food that can lead to unhealthy obsessive behaviour around food. Food Optimising – understanding which foods need to be counted and so taken under your control, and which don't – is so very liberating for slimmers who have tended to view their eating (and their stores of fat) as rushing out of control.

> TIP
> *Count Syns carefully and be realistic. If you are going to a wedding, a party or some other event and you know it will be hard to stay with a low Syn allowance for the day, estimate how many Syns you will actually need. If it's 50, then accept it. Aim to use your 50 Syns and enjoy them. Next day, get back to your normal lower allowance. It works. It works because you stay aware and you stay in control. All too often slimmers feel so guilty after eating 'too much' that they give up their healthy-eating goals altogether, thinking 'I've blown it. I just can't do it.' And they stop counting altogether for that day, that week, that month. Fifty Syns can be an awful lot less than what happens when you stop counting altogether.*

Food Optimising with Syns

• Choose between 5 and 15 Syns a day, depending on how much weight you have to lose and how fast you want to lose it. Don't forget, around 500g-1kg/1-2lb a week on average is the safest rate of weight loss. Any more and you could seriously diminish your levels of

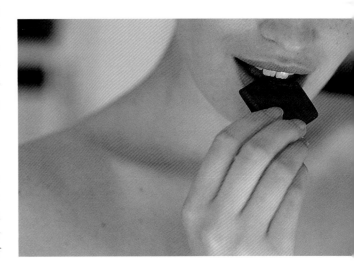

Fibre-rich foods carry more texture – which means more chewing – and that's a bonus appetite satisfier.

lean tissue and in so doing reduce your metabolic rate – and that means it gets harder to keep that weight off for good.

• If you overrun your Syn allowance, just keep counting – no need to feel guilty. No need to punish yourself by overcompensating later.

• Not sure how many Syns in a food? See the introductory list on page 43.

• Doing without Syns could mean you're being too rigid. Including your favourite treats means you're more likely to stick with it. Relax. Food Optimising is a new way to eat for life so that the weight never returns to haunt you.

Wise with fibre

Fibre is an extremely valuable part of any healthy diet. It can help protect against many illnesses, including heart disease (by reducing cholesterol), bowel diseases such as cancer of the colon and the unpleasant condition of constipation. As we've said, fibre-rich foods add bulk and are among the most effective appetite satisfiers. Food Optimising makes the most of the most fibre-rich foods for the least amount of calories.

Value for calories – that's what Food Optimising is all about! The most satisfying and nutritious foods for the least calories, without having to even think calories ever again.

Food Optimising with fibre

• Choose F or FF marked foods from the charts on pages 42-3.
• Vary the sorts of fibre you choose for maximum health benefits.
• Add beans to snacks.
• Eat at least five portions of fruit and vegetables a day – these are a good source of fibre and an immensely powerful protection against many diseases.
• Eat wholemeal varieties of bread.
• Add lentils to casseroles.
• Breakfast on a wholegrain cereal.
• If you've been eating a fibre-poor diet, increase fibre-rich foods slowly.
• Drink plenty of water when increasing fibre intake.

Are you ready to start Food Optimising?

The following chapters have menus and recipes for you to get started on and we know you'll enjoy the variety and the feeling of losing weight comfortably. Here are some tips to ensure your success.

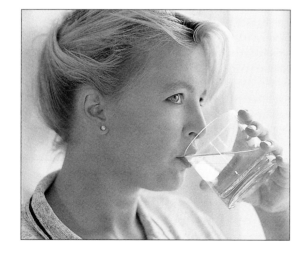

• Be realistic – gradual and small changes made to your eating habits are easier to keep up long-term.

• Set yourself mini-targets, such as 1.5kg/3lb, then 4kg/half a stone, etc. Reaching a mini-target for weight loss can be a great motivation booster and will encourage you to continue with your planned weight loss. Reward yourself when you reach your mini-target with a special treat that's not food related.

• Set motivating goals for yourself, e.g. being able to walk upstairs without getting breathless, being able to join in activities with your children, fitting into clothes that are several sizes smaller.

• Use lots of flavourings such as fresh herbs, garlic, lemon juice, chilli, and Worcestershire sauce. These will help you to lessen your reliance on all those higher-calorie sauces.

• Make a list of the reasons why you hate being overweight, why you want to slim and what you look forward to when you've lost weight. Keep it handy and look at it whenever your motivation flags.

• Boost the variety in your meals. Lack of variety is a great slimming tripwire.

• Don't ban any foods from your slimming plan. Always include your favourite foods as part of your healthy balanced diet.

• Whatever you do, don't punish yourself or try to make up for it later. A cycle of restriction and bingeing is very uncomfortable as a diet method and can't be sustained. Just put yesterday behind you and get straight back on track with your plan.

• Set increased activity goals. This doesn't necessarily mean joining a gym – it means adding extra movement into your everyday life. Research shows that people who simply fidget a lot keep their weight more stable than those who sit entirely motionless. So even as small a move as a fidget can help create a leaner body. Slimming World's Body Magic programme is designed to help you build activity into your everyday life in a way that works for you, and that you can stick to in the long term. Stairs are exercise, so are dancing, walking and gardening. Add a couple more sessions of normal activity into your daily routines. Go slowly, and aim to sustain whatever activity you have chosen.

It's time to Optimise – enjoy it and good luck!

• Support could make a crucial difference to your success. Tell chosen trusted friends or family that you're Food Optimising and that it's important to you. Ask for support and encouragement. If you explain that you are fully committed to losing weight, then they may be less likely to tease and tempt you with foods you don't want. Your local Slimming World offers a very special brand of support, so, if your motivation dwindles, we'd be delighted to welcome you there.

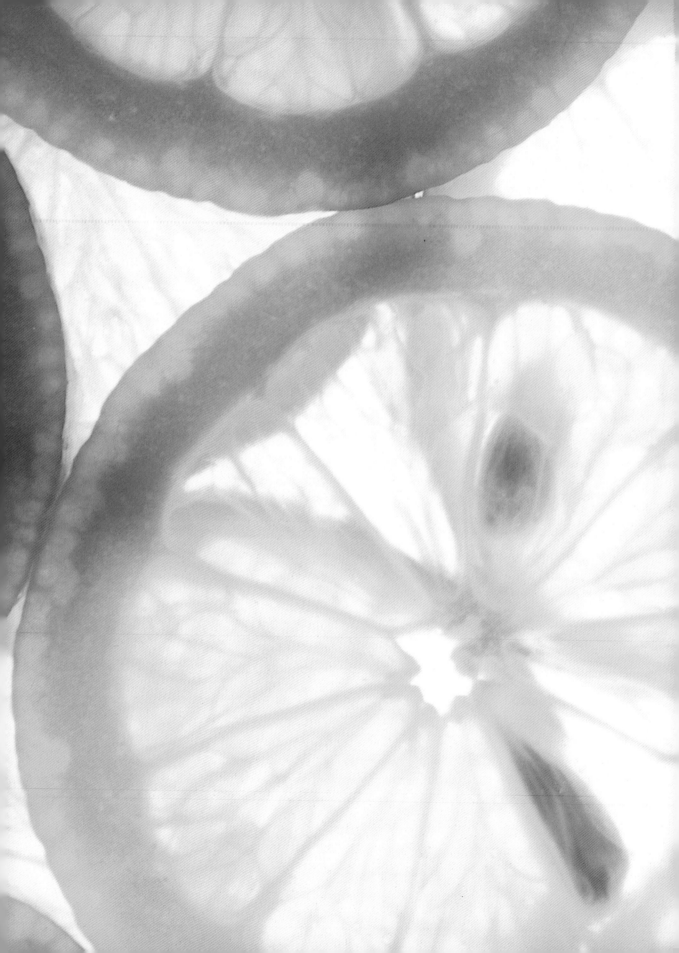

chapter 3

food optimising menus

3 Food Optimising Menus

The chances are that you are eating fairly erratically, adjusting day to day according to the demands of your busy life. And it's more than likely your current way of eating is doing your shape no favours.

Take a week or two to follow the super, tasty and varied menus given on pages 34-41 – these form a great start to Food Optimising and incorporate many of the recipes provided in this book. Although you will need to plan your shopping, you'll be thrilled to find that Food Optimising works and that you can lose weight as easily as this. We have included some of the recipes from this book in the menus. However, if you want to use a different recipe, simply check the Syn values shown for each recipes on the chart on pages 218-221.

The menus will help you to understand the variety of meals that are possible with Food Optimising. They also ensure that you have enough good, nourishing food to keep you healthy and enable you to lose weight over a period of time.

Here's how to use Food Optimising menus most effectively:

• Decide whether you wish to have a Green or Original day and stick to that choice all day. You can make every day a Green day or include some Original days too. Within the Green menus we have included meat-free choices suitable for vegetarians.

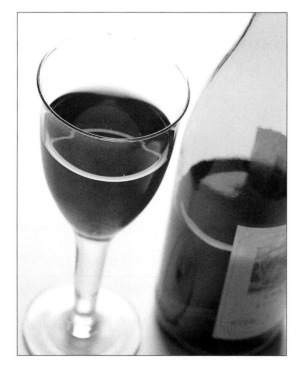

• Pick one breakfast, one lunch and one dinner from your chosen set.

• Here's the fun bit – you can choose around 10 to 15 Syns-worth of food from the Syns list following the menus (page 43). Some Food Optimisers find they lose weight best on 5 Syns, others on 20 Syns. On some days, you might find you need to use 30, if perhaps you are going out or celebrating. In general, we find 10 Syns a day is a good rule of thumb for effective weight loss.

• Check the foods on the menus that are marked in bold. These can be eaten freely without any weighing or measuring at all. Fill up on these foods when you feel peckish. You can also turn to the Free Food list at the end of the menus (see page 42-43) and select other Free Foods to enjoy whenever you want and in whatever quantity you want.

Maximise your healthy eating

• Eat at least five portions of fresh fruit and vegetables every day. Frozen and canned vegetables can also be used.

• Trim any visible fat off meat and remove any skin from poultry.

• Vary your choices as much as possible to ensure the widest range of nutrients in your diet.

• Eat at least two portions of fish a week, of which one should be oily fish.

• Aim to keep your salt intake to no more than 6g a day (about 1 level teaspoon). As well as limiting the amount of table salt you add to food, watch out for salt added to manufactured foods and sauces. Try flavouring foods with herbs and spices instead.

• Remember the latest recommendations regarding intake of fluids, which is to aim for 6-8 cups, mugs or glasses of any type of fluid per day (excluding alcohol).

• Choose a milk allowance each day from the following:
350ml/12fl oz skimmed milk
250ml/8fl oz semi-skimmed milk
175ml/6fl oz whole milk
250ml/8fl oz calcium-enriched soya milk, sweetened or unsweetened.

• Or if you prefer cheese rather than milk, choose a cheese allowance from the following:
28g/1oz Cheddar
28g/1oz Edam
28g/1oz Gouda
42g/1½oz Mozzarella
42g/1½oz reduced-fat Cheddar/Cheshire
2x20g triangles Original Dairylea

• Drink black tea, coffee (sweetened with artificial sweetener) and low-calorie drinks freely and use fat-free French or vinaigrette-style salad dressings freely.

When you have experienced the pleasure of Food Optimising on your plate you will want to make your own menus. You can do this with the complete Food Optimising system (see page 221 for further information).

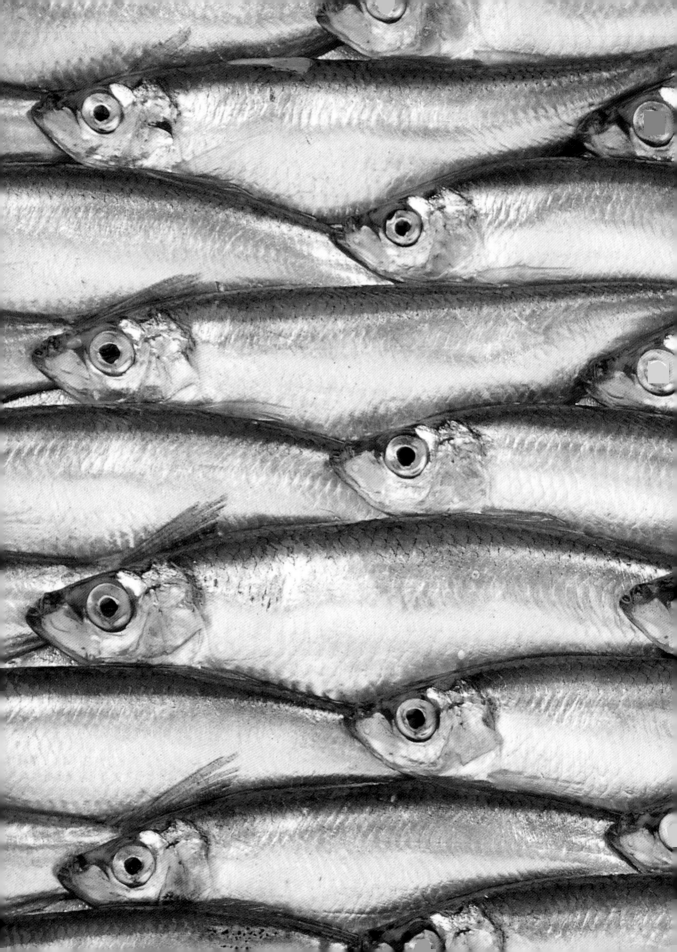

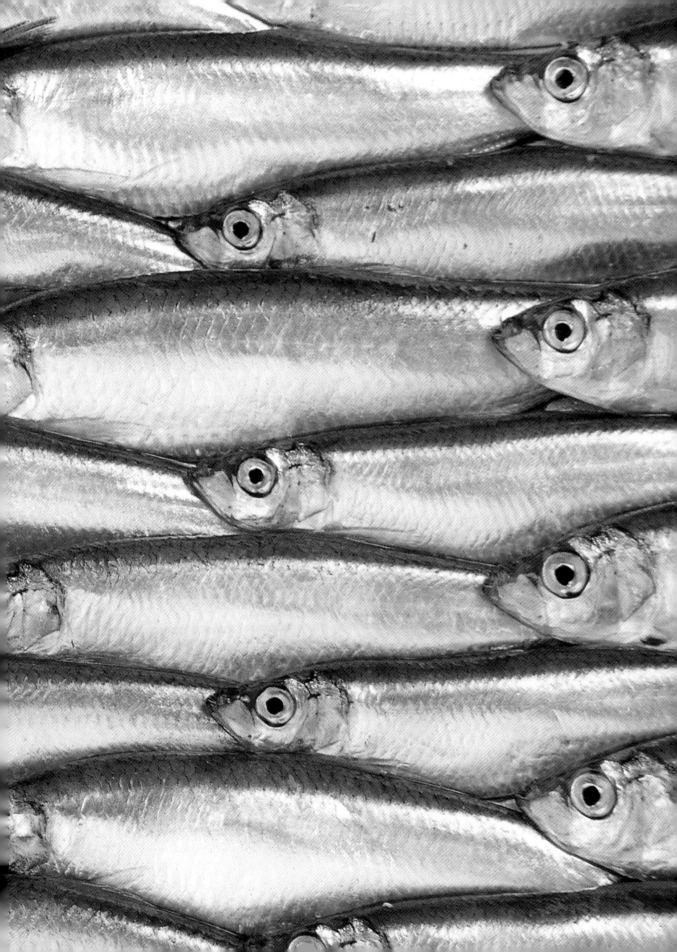

Green menus

1. Fresh **melon** wedges followed by 28g/1oz Shredded Wheat Honey Nut served with milk from allowance topped with fresh **strawberries**.

2. Two small slices wholemeal bread, toasted and topped with **baked beans** in tomato sauce. Plus an **apple** and **banana**.

3. Fresh **grapefruit** followed by two small slices of wholemeal bread toasted and topped with 28g/1oz Cheddar cheese from the allowance topped with a dash of **Worcestershire sauce**.

4. 85g/3oz grilled lean bacon (approximately three rashers), poached **egg**, grilled **tomatoes** and **mushrooms**. Plus a **peach**.

5. Two Weetabix served with milk from the allowance followed by a **banana** and some **grapes**.

6. Two small slices wholemeal bread, toasted and topped with scrambled or poached **eggs**. Plus a **fresh fruit salad** topped with a **Müllerlight yogurt**.

7. 28g/1oz Kellogg's Chocolate Wheats topped with sliced fresh **banana** and served with milk from the allowance. Plus an **orange**.

8. 340g/12oz apricots, canned in juice followed by an **omelette** filled with 28g/1oz grated Cheddar cheese from the allowance and sliced **mushrooms** served with **baked beans** in tomato sauce and grilled **tomatoes**.

9. 28g/1oz bran flakes topped with **raspberries** and served with milk from the allowance. Plus an

apple or **pear** and a **satsuma**.

10. Two small slices of wholemeal bread, toasted and topped with plum **tomatoes** and **mushrooms**. Plus **plums** or a **peach**.

11. Yogurt crunch made with **very low fat natural yogurt**, 28g/1oz Jordans Luxury Muesli and sliced **kiwi**: layer the kiwi, muesli and yogurt in a tall glass finishing with a sprinkling of muesli and a slice of kiwi. Plus 1 Ryvita Wholegrain Crackerbread topped with sliced **banana**.

12. 42g/1½oz grilled kippers with scrambled **egg** and grilled **tomatoes**, followed by an **orange**.

13. Half cantaloupe **melon** filled with fresh **raspberries** or **grapes**. Plus 42g/1½oz Bran Buds served with milk from the allowance.

14. Baked beans, grilled **tomatoes**, poached **mushrooms** and poached **eggs** served with two small slices of wholemeal bread, toasted. Plus a **banana**.

LUNCHES

1. Chinese Vegetable Salad (see recipe on page 167) followed by 283g/10oz blackberries, stewed without sugar topped with **very low-fat natural yogurt**.

2. Jacket potato filled with 42g/1½oz reduced fat Cheddar cheese, grated and chopped **spring onions** served with lots of **salad**. Plus an **apple** or **banana**.

3. Jacket potato filled with 113g/4oz tuna,

canned in brine, and **sweetcorn** served with **radicchio, endive, radishes**, cherry **tomatoes** and fresh **orange** segments.

4. Mixed Bean Salad (see recipe on page 174) served with two small slices of wholemeal bread. Plus some **plums**.

5. 142g/5oz haddock or cod served with **Slimming World's Syn-free Chips** (see recipe on page 156) and mushy **peas**. Plus an **apple**.

6. 57g/2oz wholemeal crusty roll filled with sliced **egg** and **watercress** followed by fresh **strawberries** topped with **very low-fat natural yogurt**.

7. 85g/3oz smoked salmon topped with **very low-fat natural cottage cheese** and freshly chopped **chives** and then rolled up, served with new **potatoes** cooked with fresh **mint** and lots of **salad**.

8. Two small slices of wholemeal bread, toasted and topped with canned **spaghetti** and scrambled **egg**. Plus a **pear** and **banana.**

9. Pasta salad made with **pasta** shapes, cherry **tomatoes**, chopped **peppers, cucumber, sweetcorn** and freshly chopped **basil** mixed with **quark** flavoured with freshly chopped **garlic**. Plus a 227g/8oz baked apple topped with 113g/4oz blackberries, stewed without sugar and **very low-fat natural fromage frais**.

10. 57g/2oz lean roast beef served with mashed **potato, swede**, **peas, leeks** and **carrots**.

Followed by a fresh fruit cocktail made with chopped fresh **pineapple, peach** and **kiwi fruit**.

11. Couscous salad made with **couscous, cucumber, borlotti beans**, 20 cashew nuts and freshly chopped **mint** mixed together with **fat-free vinaigrette-style salad dressing**. Plus a bunch of **grapes**.

12. Two small slices of wholemeal bread, toasted and topped with **baked beans** in tomato sauce and 28g/1oz grated Cheddar cheese from the allowance. Plus a **pear** and **plums**.

13. Sandwich made with two small slices of wholemeal bread filled with **mixed green leaves** and homemade coleslaw: finely shredded red and green **cabbage**, grated **carrot**, chopped **apple** and **spring onions** mixed with **very low-fat natural yogurt** and seasoning. Plus a bunch of **grapes**.

14. Spicy Cajun Chicken Salad (see recipe on page 178). Plus a wedge of **melon.**

DINNERS

1. Mushroom Stroganoff (see recipe on page 141) served with basmati **rice, broccoli** and **green beans**. Plus some **grapes** and **plums**.

2. Indian-style Rice and Split Peas (see recipe on page 134). Plus a selection of fresh **berries** topped with **very low-fat natural fromage frais** flavoured with **vanilla**.

3. Tagliatelle mixed with **quark**, freshly

chopped **basil** and **black pepper** topped with cooked sliced **courgettes** and diced **aubergine**. Followed by **Oriental Green Fruit Salad** (see recipe on page 192).

4. Curried Lentil and Quorn Burgers (see recipe on page 129) served with a jacket **potato** and lots of **salad**. Plus an **apple** and **orange**

5. Baked Couscous Pudding with Chunky Chilli Vegetable Sauce (see recipe on page 131) served with new **potatoes**, butternut **squash, leeks** and **cabbage**. Plus a **Müllerlight yogurt**.

6. Mixed Root Vegetable Soup (see recipe on page 70) followed by **Spanish-style Tortilla** (see recipe on page 145) served with a selection of **vegetables** or a mixed **salad**. Plus a bowl of fresh tropical fruit salad made with chopped **mango, kiwi fruit** and **papaya**.

7. Corn on the cob followed by **Root Vegetable and Lentil Casserole** (see recipe on page 142) served with mashed **potato** and a selection of **green vegetables**. Plus sliced **kiwi** and seedless **grapes**.

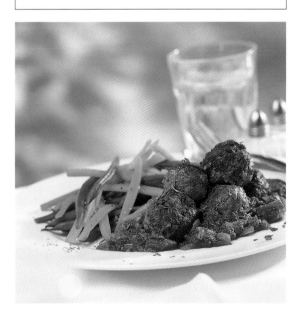

8. Vegetable crudités: strips of **carrot, cucumber, baby sweetcorn** and **cauliflower florets** served with a tzatziki dip (**very low-fat natural yogurt**, mixed with chopped **cucumber**, crushed **garlic**, chopped **mint** and seasoning). Followed by **Quorn chunks** served with **Spicy Red Roast Vegetables** (see recipe on page 160). Plus a **banana**.

9. Omelette filled with chopped **peppers**, red **onions, sweetcorn** and **quark** served with a jacket **potato** and lots of **salad**. Plus half a canteloupe **melon** filled with **raspberries**.

10. Pasta topped with a chunky pasta sauce made with chopped **tomatoes, celery, courgettes, mushrooms**, mixed **peppers, sweetcorn, onion, garlic** and **herbs**. Plus an **apple** and **satsuma**.

11. Ratatouille with Eggs (see recipe on page 144) served with freshly cooked **rice** and a crisp **salad**. Followed by **very low-fat natural fromage frais** mixed with sliced **banana** and **vanilla**.

12. Macaroni Cheese Stuffed Peppers (see recipe on page 122) served with a large mixed **salad** and boiled **rice**. Plus a pot of **very low-fat natural yogurt** and a **pear**.

13. Vegetable stir-fry: **broccoli** and **cauliflower** florets, chopped **carrots**, mixed **peppers, spring onions**, button **mushrooms, beansprouts** and **water chestnuts** stir fried with **garlic, herbs** and **soy sauce** served on a bed of **bulgur wheat** or **couscous**. Plus an **apple**.

14. Jacket **potato** filled with mixed **beans** served with lots of mixed **salad**. Plus **strawberries** topped with **very low-fat natural fromage frais** flavoured with vanilla.

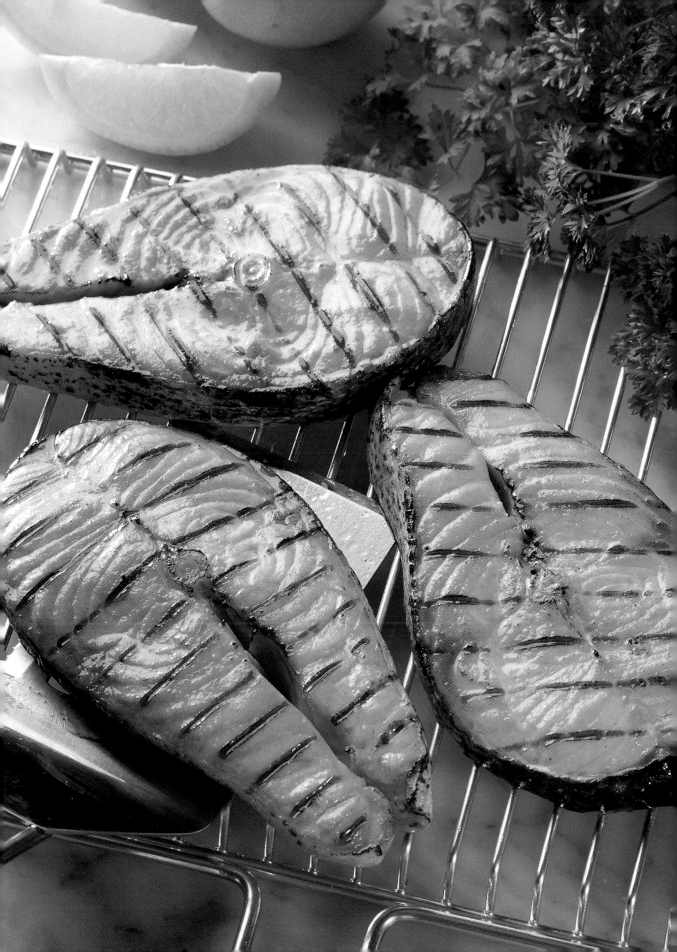

Original menus

BREAKFASTS

1. Fresh **grapefruit** plus lean grilled **gammon**, poached **egg**, grilled **tomatoes** and **mushrooms** served with two small slices of wholemeal bread, toasted.

2. Fresh **grapefruit** segments followed by two small slices wholemeal bread filled with grilled lean **bacon**.

3. Fresh **apricots**, chopped and topped with **very low-fat natural fromage frais** or **yogurt** followed by grilled lean **bacon**, poached **egg** and 142g/5oz baked beans in tomato sauce.

4. 28g/1oz porridge oats made with milk from the allowance sprinkled with **cinnamon** followed by grilled **kippers** served with scrambled **egg**.

5. Two Weetabix served with milk from the allowance. Follow this with an **orange** or **pear**.

6. 42g/1½oz All Bran/Fibre Plus topped with a sliced **banana** and served with milk from the allowance.

7. 142g/5oz prunes canned in juice and **omelette** (cooked with no fat) filled with lean **ham** and **mushrooms**.

8. A slice of **melon** followed by boiled **eggs** served with two small slices of wholemeal toast cut into soldiers.

9. A slice of **melon** followed by 28g/1oz Shredded Wheat Fruitful served with milk from the allowance.

10. Two small slices wholemeal toast topped with poached **eggs**. Plus a **banana**.

11. Grilled lean **bacon**, scrambled **egg**, grilled **tomatoes** and **mushrooms**. Plus 71g/2½oz dried apricots.

12. Two small slices wholemeal toast topped with plum **tomatoes** with a dash of **Worcestershire sauce**. Plus a **peach** or **nectarine**.

13. Fresh **orange** and **grapefruit** segments followed by two small slices wholemeal toast topped with **Marmite**.

14. Selection of fresh or frozen **berries** topped with **very low-fat natural fromage frais** or **yogurt**. Plus 28g/1oz Alpen served with milk from the allowance.

LUNCHES

1. **Salmon** fillet baked in the oven with **coriander** and **lemon juice** served with a large mixed **salad** and 227g/8oz baked potato (raw weight) followed by **grapes**.

2. Roast Beef with Mexican-style Coleslaw (see recipe on page 152) served with two small slices of wholemeal bread. Plus a **banana** and **pear**.

3. Smoked **cod** served with scrambled **egg** and grilled **tomatoes** and two small slices wholemeal bread followed by a **Müllerlight Yogurt** and an **apple**.

4. Prawns served on a bed of **mixed salad**

leaves and **asparagus** topped with a sprinkling of **lemon juice** and fresh **parsley** served with two small slices wholemeal bread followed by a **banana** and **grapes**.

5. Large mixed salad served with **tuna** canned in brine and 113g/4oz red kidney beans followed by fresh **strawberries** and cubes of **melon**.

6. Roast **chicken** breast served with 227g/8oz jacket potato (raw weight), together with **broccoli, carrots** and **mange tout** followed by a **pear**.

7. 227g/8oz jacket potato (raw weight) filled with **very low-fat natural cottage cheese** and chopped **spring onions** served with lots of **salad**. Plus chopped **apple** and **orange** segments topped with **very low-fat natural fromage frais**.

8. Pork and Herb Meatballs with Ratatouille Sauce (see recipe on page 104) served on a bed of 100g/4oz wholemeal spaghetti (boiled weight) followed by rings of fresh **pineapple**.

9. Two small slices wholemeal bread filled with **smoked salmon** and **quark** served with a mixed **salad**. Plus **kiwi fruit** and **plums**.

10. 57g/2oz wholemeal crusty roll filled with **chicken** and **salad** followed by a **Müllerlight Yogurt** and a **banana**.

11. Stir-fried Summer Vegetables (see recipe on page 164). Plus 255g/9oz raspberries, stewed without sugar.

12. Lean roast **beef** served with 198g/7oz new potatoes boiled in skins, together with **carrots,** thin **green beans** and **cabbage** followed by fresh **strawberries** and **blueberries**.

13. Seafood Niçoise Salad (see recipe on page 175). Plus fresh **raspberries** topped with **very low-fat natural yogurt**.

14. BLT sandwich made with two small slices of wholemeal bread filled with grilled lean **bacon, lettuce** and sliced **tomato**. Plus an **apple** and bunch of **grapes**.

DINNERS

1. Lean fillet **steak** tossed in crushed black **peppercorns** and then grilled until cooked to preference, served with **baby whole sweetcorn, sugar snap peas** and **asparagus**. Plus fresh fruit salad, e.g. chopped **apple, banana** and **peach**.

2. Grilled **mackerel** served with lots of **salad** followed by a **Müllerlight Yogurt**.

3. Garlic Chicken and Vegetable Pot Roast (see recipe on page 90) served with **leeks** and **cauliflower**.

4. Cajun Griddled Fish (see recipe on page 110) served with lots of **salad** followed by fresh **melon**.

5. Lean **pork** steaks, grilled and served with **swede, cabbage** and **carrots**. Followed by **Pineapple and Mint Cocktail** (see recipe on page 190).

6. Prawns sprinkled with **paprika** served on a bed of crisp **lettuce** and **cucumber** followed by a **chicken** breast, grilled or baked, served with **red cabbage,** thin **green beans** and **butternut squash**. Plus a bowl of **raspberries, blackberries** and **blueberries** topped with **very low-fat natural fromage frais**.

7. Roast Lamb with a Curried Crust (see recipe on page 98) served with **sugar snap peas, carrots** and **broccoli**. Plus a **Mullerlight Yogurt**.

8. Omelette filled with diced lean **ham** and **onion** served with heaps of **salad**. Plus **satsumas**.

9. Lean **gammon** steak, grilled, topped with fresh **pineapple** chunks served with **salad leaves**, cherry **tomatoes, cucumber, spring onions** and grated **carrot**. Plus a **banana**.

10. Honeydew melon, followed by fresh **tuna steak**, chargrilled and served with **asparagus, carrots** and **courgettes**. Plus fresh **mango** and sliced seedless **grapes**.

11. Gazpacho with Prawns (see recipe on page 67) followed by **lemon sole** or **plaice** baked with fresh **lime** wedges served on a bed of **spinach** with thin **green beans** and **mange tout**.

12. Insalata di Mare (see recipe on page 74). Plus a bowl of **strawberries** topped with **very low-fat natural fromage frais**.

13. Kleftico-style Lamb Steaks (see recipe on page 96) served with baby **leeks, asparagus** and Savoy **cabbage**.

14. Monkfish and Bacon Kebabs (see recipe on page 115) served with heaps of **salad**. Plus a bowl of chopped **kiwi** and fresh **pineapple**.

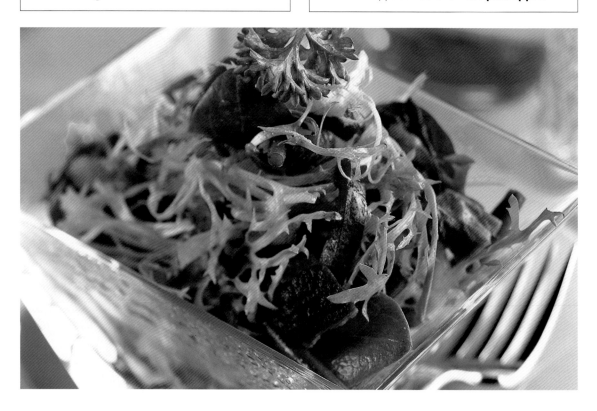

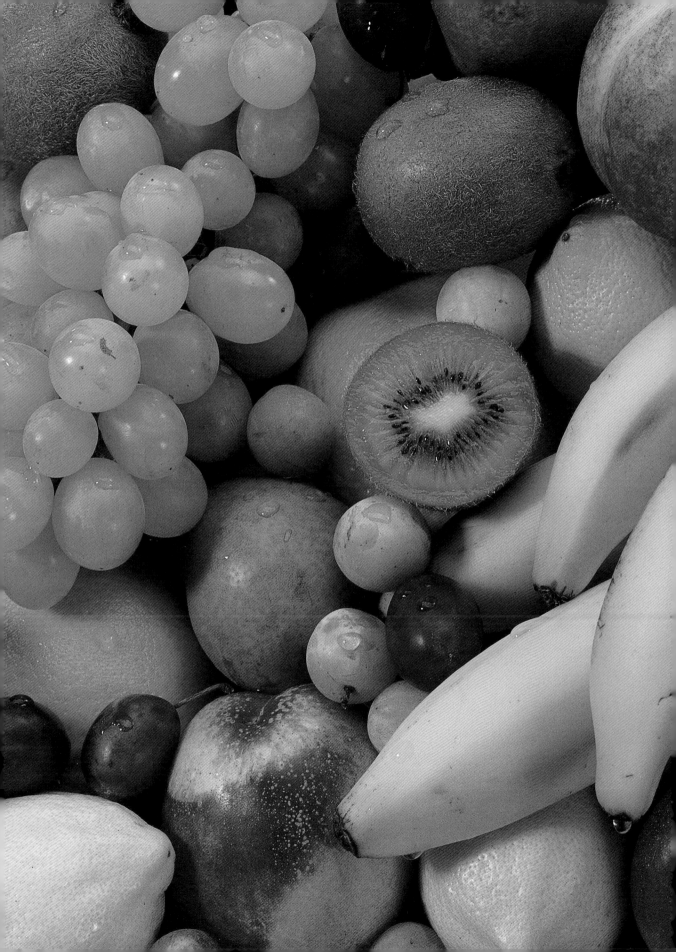

free foods and treat selections

• We have listed some of our Free Foods here. For the full list, you will need to become a Slimming World member (see page 221).

• Foods marked with an S symbol will give your weight loss a boost. Choosing foods marked with a SS symbol will give your weight loss an even bigger boost.

• Foods marked with an F will give you extra fibre and those marked with FF will give you an even richer helping of fibre.

• Foods marked H will keep you healthy and those marked HH are vital to your health and need to be included every day.

Green Day Free Foods

All vegetables are classed as a Free Food when on a Green day.

Broccoli		S	HH
Celeriac	F	S	HH
Potatoes			HH
Rice			H
Dried pasta			H
Buckwheat			H
Couscous			H
Baked beans	F	SS	H
Chick peas	F		H
Red kidney beans	FF	S	H
Soya beans	FF		H
Lentils	F	S	H
Peas	F	S	H
Quorn	F	S	H
Eggs			
Tofu			
Bananas			HH
Apples		S	HH

Peaches		S	HH
Oranges		S	HH
Grapefruit		SS	HH
Strawberries		SS	HH
Pineapple		S	HH
Very low-fat natural yogurt			H
Very low-fat natural fromage frais			H

Original Day Free Foods

Not all vegetables are Free Foods on Original days: choose from only those listed here for a Syn-free day.

Artichokes	F		HH
Asparagus		S	HH
Aubergine		S	HH
Baby whole sweetcorn		S	HH
Beans – French, runner		S	HH
Beetroot		S	HH
Broccoli		S	HH
Brussels sprouts	F		HH
Cabbage		S	HH
Carrots		S	HH
Cauliflower		S	HH
Courgettes		S	HH
Leeks		S	HH
Mushrooms		S	HH
Onions		S	HH
Spinach		S	HH
Squash		S	HH
Swede		S	HH
Quorn	F	S	H
Chicken, all fat and skin removed		S	H
Turkey, all fat and skin removed		S	H
Cod		SS	H
Crab		S	H
Haddock		SS	H
Kippers			H
Mackerel (not smoked)			H

Pilchards		H
Plaice	SS	H
Prawns	S	H
Salmon		H
Sole	S	H
Caviare		H
Bacon		
Beef		
Ham		
Lamb		
Pork		
Eggs		
Tofu		
Apples	S	HH
Bananas		HH
Oranges	S	HH
Grapes		HH
Pineapple	S	HH
Strawberries	SS	HH
Very low-fat natural yogurt		H
Very low-fat natural fromage frais		H

Treat selection

We have listed here a selection of Syn values for foods that you can enjoy every day. A list of nearly 40,000 Syn values is available from Slimming World (for further information see page 221).

ALCOHOL

25ml/1fl oz measure of any spirit	2½
142ml/¼pt glass of wine	5
284ml/½pt lager/beer	5
284ml/½pt cider	5

BISCUITS

Custard cream	3
Digestive	3½
Jammie Dodger	4
Morning Coffee	1
Chocolate finger	1½
Rich tea	2
Jaffa cake/ginger nut	2½
Shortcake	2½

CRISPS (per standard bag)

French fries	4½
Quavers	5½
Wotsits	5½
Ryvita Minis	5
Standard potato crisps (per 28g/1oz)	7½

CHOCOLATE AND SWEETS (per standard bar/tube/bag unless stated)

Fun-size bars	5
Curly Wurly	6
Two-finger Kit Kat	5½
Fruit Gums	8½
Fudge	6
Milky Bar	3½
Penguin bar	5½

CAKES (individual, average)

Custard tart	12
Jam doughnut	12½
Ring doughnut	12
Danish pastry	19
Mince pie	11
Eccles cake	9½
Mr Kipling Cake Bites	3½
Mr Kipling Country/Lemon Slices	6

SAUCES AND SPREADS

Gravy made from granules, made with no fat, 4tbsp	1
Reduced calorie mayonnaise, 1 level tbsp	2½
Custard made with skimmed milk, 2 level tbsp	1½
Margarine/spread low-fat variety, 28g/1oz	5½
Olive oil/any oil, 1 level tbsp	6

NUTS

Peanuts/almonds, fresh/roast/dry roast, 28g/1oz	8½
Cashew nuts, shelled, 28g/1oz	8
Walnuts, shelled, 28g/1oz	9½

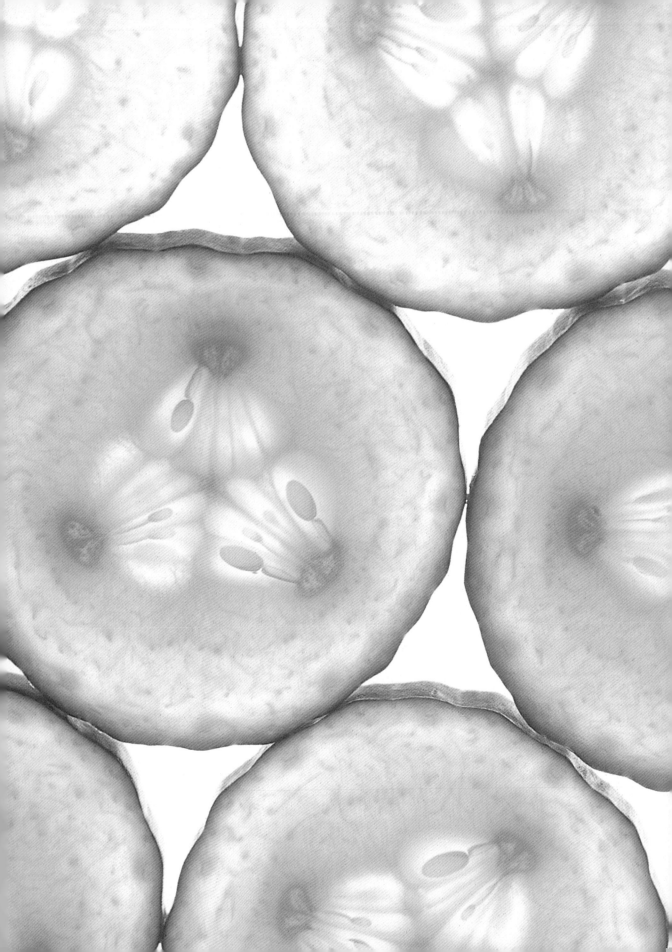

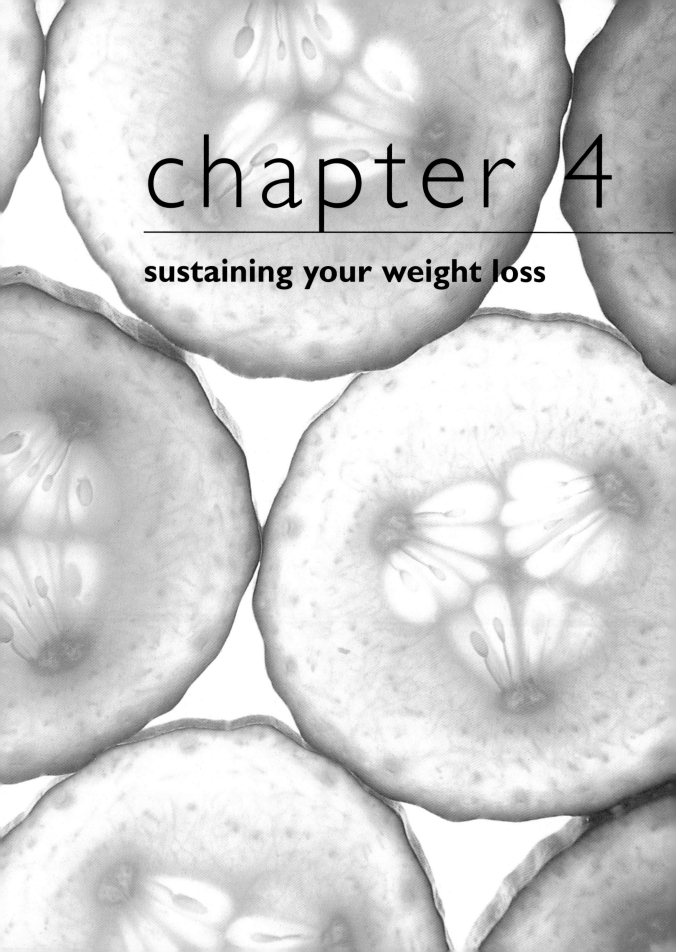

chapter 4

sustaining your weight loss

4 Sustaining your Weight Loss

Underpinning Slimming World is a basic belief, a philosophy, born of a deep understanding of the burden of excess weight. It's about respect and holding overweight people in high regard. There's no contemptuous humiliation, no disapproval, no put downs of even the most subtle kind. Instead there is warmth, understanding, praise and support.

Beauty confidence

If being slim were the only way to be beautiful, most of the population of most countries would look dull, dowdy and depressed. But it is blindingly obvious as you walk through the streets of any major city that beauty is a constellation of factors clinging to certain people and not others. Those beautiful people – and they are not rare – have understood their personal worth, and expressed it in their way of walking, talking, dressing, interacting with the world about them.

Each one of us has a personal, unique and striking beauty but we don't always realise it. Life sometimes damages our sense of individual beauty. Fashion and our culture can rob all but the thinnest of our sense of worth.

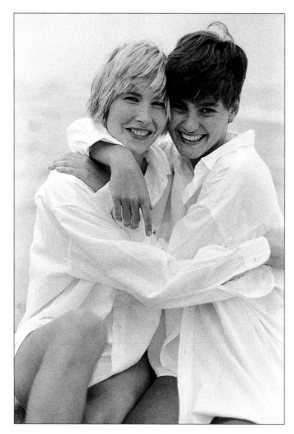

The beauty of you

If you have lost the art of knowing your own beauty, you'll need support to get your beauty-confidence back. Start to listen to what loving friends and family say about you – really take notice. We usually dismiss compliments, even when they regularly flow in our direction. It isn't 'cool' to praise ourselves, but actually it's very cool indeed to take a compliment with good grace, accepting it for what it is.

At Slimming World compliments, giving and receiving, are standard fare. In fact, they flow naturally from our special brand of group therapy. It's called Individual Motivation and Group Experience (IMAGE) Therapy and it enables a group of slimmers to work on the real needs – and acknowledge the real achievements and gifts – of every member.

Slimming is about achieving a tough goal as it requires working through a real change in lifestyle, and the glow you get from that translates into beauty very easily indeed. People around you, because they appreciate the value of the pounds you've lost each week, want to applaud you – and they do. The whole experience is like a warm blanket that wraps itself around you, comforting and strong. In just a few short minutes, every single person has the combined power and sup-

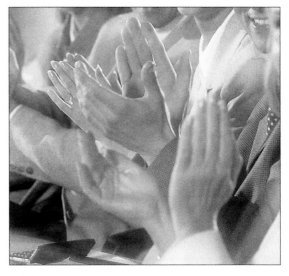

port of the whole group working for them. And the focus is not just on you but on your future, not your past. It's like a magic spotlight that shines and illuminates the way forward in a completely positive way so that when motivation starts to flag, instead of sliding down the slippery slope into hopelessness you find your footing again.

If you've put on weight in between groups, rather than a tut tut when you come back to group you'll get a pat on the back. Why? Because we know what it's like. You didn't have a very good week and you knew you'd probably put on a little weight. You could have stayed at home and hoped to do better next week. Of course, you'd probably have slipped further. But you didn't do that. Even though you weren't feeling too good about yourself and didn't really want anyone to know that you'd gained a pound, you came anyway to refuel your motivation and get the help you needed. That took a great deal of courage and a lot of common sense. That's why you deserve praise and you'll get it.

At Slimming World, we understand that guilt happens around eating and part of our mission is to help you know that YOU are not guilty of any wrongdoing. YOU are an able, effective, beautiful and worthwhile person and YOU are able to control your life and your weight. It's really worth remembering that overeating is simply taking in more energy (calories) than we use up. That can happen *Fat is not a moral issue* if our activity levels have reduced over the years as our intake of fat-rich foods has increased slightly. The imbalance can be small, but over a period of months or years, quite devastating in terms of weight gain.

To regulate your responses to life and to achieve your weight loss goals, there are some techniques that Slimming World can share with you. After forty years of working with every type of weight loss problem and every variety of slimmer, our techniques are tried and tested.

Making decisions

The key to staying in control of your weight loss plan is making the right decisions. Right decisions are those that will, sooner or later, lead us to achieving our goal. They are small everyday decisions that affect every action we take, such as deciding to weigh yourself once a week rather

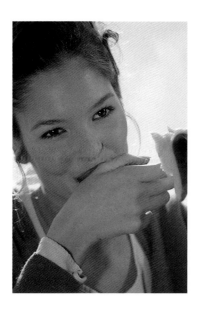

than every day. But even before we step on the scales, making the right decision about our lifestyle, food, each meal, each change in a pattern of behaviour becomes a positive reinforcement of our sense of self worth.

Decision making also gives us a positive opportunity to get what we want. The opportunity lies in the many, many everyday things we do without actually making a real decision. We say yes to a chocolate without thinking. We have a sticky toffee pudding because everyone is raving about it. We don't think those acts through. They happen so fast, either impulsively or out of sheer habit, that we are virtually unaware of there being a choice about it.

But there is a choice, and becoming aware of the value of food, through our Free Food and Syn lists, gives you the chance to make an informed choice. And the choice is always yours – because you can have the chocolate or the sticky toffee pudding, you really can. Count your Syns and choose what is worth most to you to spend your Syns on. Then enjoy your decision.

Making a real decision is all about thinking it out first. It is also about considering before acting. Good decisions belong to you – they are absolutely your choice.

Here are two positive decisions you could make to help you in general:
• Decide to focus on the fact that in reality you are losing weight a lot quicker than you gained it.
• Decide that to lose even a single pound on a regular basis is something to be proud of. It shows you are tenacious and committed, without being obsessive.

Smaller is still beautiful

We learned at Slimming World years ago to adapt that old saying small is beautiful. Aiming for a very small size, a far lower weight, a drastically reduced quantity of food, is fraught with danger.

The positive approach that we know works is to take small steps, to set small goals, to appreciate small wonders for the big achievements they are. That's why we developed our famous Personal Achievement Target. We don't tell you what weight you should be. It's for you to look at your overall needs and wishes and decide what weight you would like to aim for. That often means a more modest weight loss than slimmers aimed at years ago.

The health benefits of losing even 10 per cent of your bodyweight if you are very overweight are well documented and even include an increase in life expectancy. So it's really worth starting small – and who knows, you may well end up losing an amount of weight that you would have thought impossible back at the beginning of your weight loss journey.

Exercise comes into the 'start small' approach. A daily 15-minute walk round the block could help you get fit if you're not fit at all. And most of us aren't! You can aim to make that 30 minutes in a few weeks' time once you are comfortably striding out each day. Slimming World's Body Magic encourages members to introduce small amounts of exercise into their lives, which make a big difference to their weight and health in the long term.

Becoming slim

We all want to be slim. Of course, that's our motivation for eating more healthily and taking care to make healthy changes in our lifestyle.

And we are acting in a slim way while we become slim. We believe at Slimming World that we are slim in a way because if our natural, healthy, balanced self were allowed to emerge, that self would be slim. We need to tell our subconscious that we actually are slim now, because in this sense, we are.

We are only overweight in the transient, passing sense. It would be extremely useful for slimmers if the English language had a different word for the verb to be. Spanish, for example, differentiates between states of being that imply either permanence or transience. We don't distinguish between the two in the English language. So you'd describe yourself by saying 'I am tall', which is a permanent state, but also say 'I am tired', which is a transient state. How about saying 'I am slim. At the moment, I am 'overweight-ing' (being temporarily overweight)' – not very grammatical but you get the picture.

Choose to feel good

Feeling good about ourselves is a vital ingredient of permanent success. It may take time to understand that we choose how we feel. We tend to

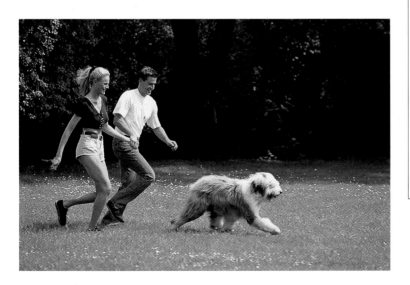

DECISION-MAKING TIPS

• Take a moment to be aware that a food decision opportunity is coming up – that's great news because it will help you get to your weight and health goal.

• Think about the value of the food offered. Is it Free? Is it worth 5 Syns? Or 40 Syns?

• If it's Free, ask yourself if you want it – just because it's Free doesn't mean it must be eaten. If you want it, wonderful, eat it and enjoy it. Don't worry about the size of your portion – it's a Free Food and you can follow your appetite.

• If it has a Syn value, ask yourself whether you want to spend the Syns on that particular food.

• If you do – accept it, eat it and enjoy it completely without guilt. You are in control.

• If you don't – you'll actually enjoy saying no and you can enjoy the feeling of being in control and the prospect of a more attractive food coming along later for you to spend your Syns on.

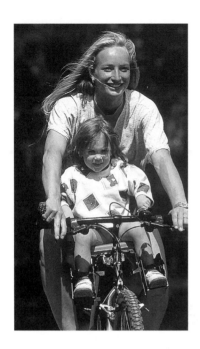

say 'he made me feel bad' or 'you made me happy' – we say it, believe it and live our lives accordingly. We become an emotional thermometer allowing our feelings to be turned up or down by someone else. Yet, others can only invite us to feel good or bad. We can decide whether or not we wish to accept the invitation. We can, therefore, be a thermostat not a thermometer. We can actually regulate and control how we feel. When we practise this on a regular basis, it can help us deal with our weight goals well.

Psychologists believe we can change our belief system in and about ourselves and achieve the level of satisfaction with ourselves that we crave. Repetition of an affirmation (a statement using only positive words about ourselves and always in the present tense) is one way to do this.

Try these affirmations:

✓ I am firm, fair and consistent in my dealings with others.

✓ I only say positive things about others.

✓ I am a loving and caring person.

✓ I respect my worth and the worth of those around me.

✓ I love being in control of my weight and my wellbeing.

✓ I am slim.

Hang on to your high

You are part of Slimming World now that you have bought this book, used our recipes and started to use some of the many techniques we have developed. We hope you already have a feel-good factor in your weight-loss plans. We hope your self-esteem is as high as it could be.

We would love you to achieve the beauty of confidence in yourself and to believe in the real slim you that exists right now. There's one very practical reason for this: you'll probably lose weight more effectively if you do. As the British Nutrition Foundation's (BNF) Task Force on Obesity (1999) said: 'Body dissatisfaction has in the past been considered to be an inevitable reaction to obesity and has rarely been targeted in treatment programmes.' We knew, many, many years ago, that this was the case and have targeted it in our groups for forty years!

The BNF goes on: 'There is now increasing recognition that [body] dissatisfaction contributes to low self-esteem and self-efficacy and could compromise compliance with treatment … Modifying body image could improve adherence to activity recommendations.' This is why Food Optimising is designed to keep you in control of your eating and your weight loss without telling you what to do, like so many fixed meal menus.

Our menus here are a guide to the world of Food Optimising. Once you understand it and you've practised it, it's a technique for you to enjoy using for a whole lifetime. It's your meal, your weight, your choice. Here are some ways to help you hang on to that high:

• *Capture your feelings at the point when your self-esteem is high. Write them down. Keep it confidential, keep it handy and turn to it when you feel your self-confidence flagging. Add anything positive you know about yourself.*

• *Add anything positive that other people have noticed that you have missed. Even when you think they are wrong, add it to the list. Chances are they are right and you have been setting yourself too high standards.*

• *Whether you realise it or not, you are superbly special. Your weight, your measurements, your size, your shape – they are not you. You are far more than that. You are kind, loving, strong, passionate and thoughtful. You are courageous, spirited and honourable. You are perfectly imperfect – which makes you just about perfect.*

If you truly decide to, you can do just about anything.

Fall in love with yourself. When you do that, those highs just last and last.

To further help you achieve weight loss, here are some questions to ask yourself before starting your weight loss campaign:

• *How much weight can I comfortably and safely lose in, say, a month?*

• *How much of that could I try to lose during the next seven days?*

• *What might stop me achieving that loss? If there are any big celebrations or problem eating times coming up, do I need to revise my week's goal?*

• *What small opportunity for activity can I see coming up during the next few days? How can I make it attractive enough to repeat it?*

These are a reflection of the sort of conversations we have in group that help slimmers clarify the few days ahead of them and come back a week later feeling satisfied. After all, it's today that we have to deal with. Even tomorrow is a long way off.

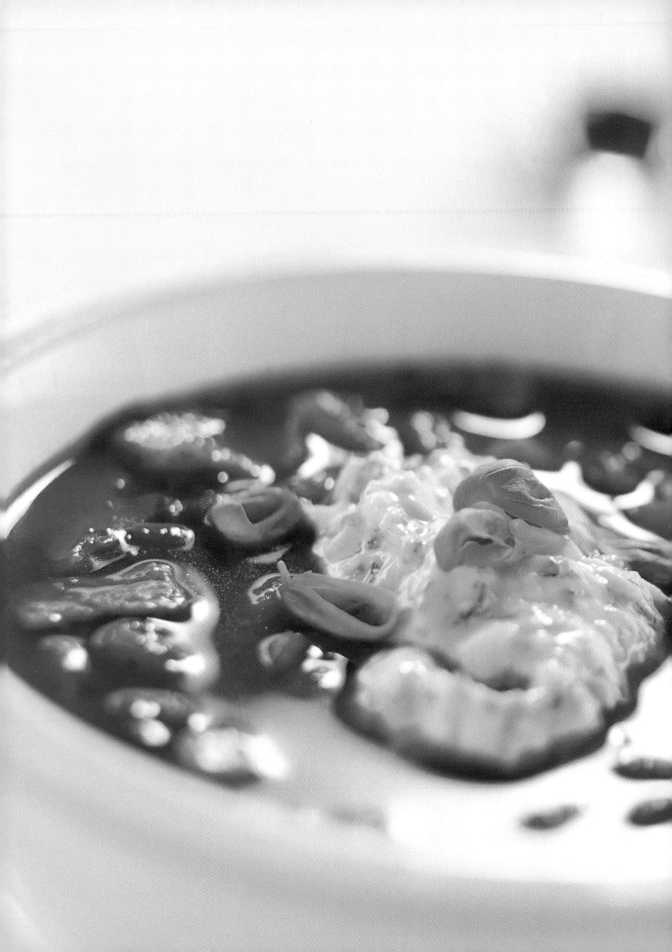

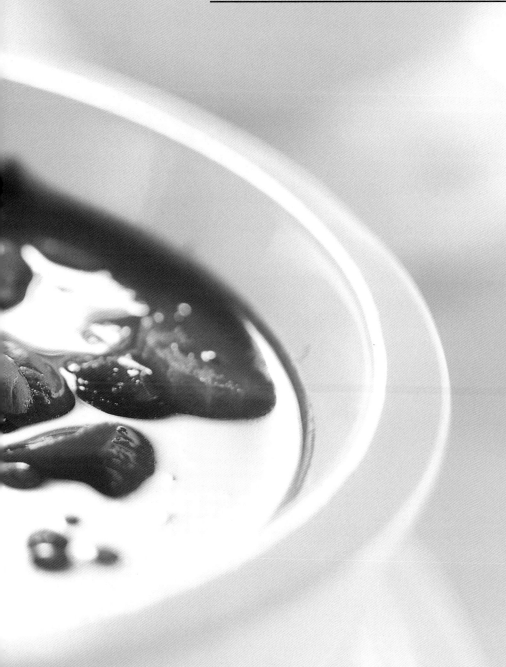

starters

mexican avocado dip

This is a lighter version of guacamole, which is usually laden with fat. The dip is full of flavour and is very colourful when served with different raw vegetables to dip into it. It is perfect to serve at parties or as a topping for baked potatoes.

Serves: 4
Preparation time: approximately
15 minutes

1 large beefsteak tomato
4 spring onions
1 small ripe avocado
2 tbsp lemon juice
113g/4oz quark skimmed milk soft cheese
2 tbsp freshly chopped coriander
Salt and freshly ground black pepper
A few drops of Tabasco sauce

1. Remove the stalk from the tomato and finely chop. Place in a bowl. Trim and finely chop the white and green parts of the spring onions and mix into the tomatoes.

2. Halve the avocado and discard the stone. Peel off the skin and mash the flesh with the lemon juice. Mix with the soft cheese.

3. Combine the avocado mixture with the chopped tomato and spring onion along with the coriander, plenty of seasoning and a few drops of Tabasco.

4. Serve with plenty of crisp vegetables like peppers, celery, radishes and cucumber to dip.

Cook's Note
Remember, Tabasco sauce is made from spicy red chillies and a few drops will add quite a lot of heat to any dish.

spinach roulade with red pepper sauce

This light sponge is perfect when you're Syn watching. It contains no flour, yet forms a deliciously moist 'cake', which is filled and rolled and served with a tangy tomato sauce. Slice it thickly for a supper or lunch, or more thinly for a starter.

Serves: 4-6
Preparation time: approximately 20 minutes
Cooking time: approximately 15 minutes

454g/1lb chopped frozen spinach, thawed
4 large eggs, separated
½ tsp ground nutmeg
Salt and freshly ground black pepper
170g/6oz roasted red pepper in brine, drained
284ml/½pt passata
227g/8oz quark skimmed milk soft cheese
4 tbsp very low-fat natural fromage frais
2 tbsp freshly chopped chives
2 level tbsp freshly grated Parmesan cheese

1. Preheat the oven to 220°C/425°G/Gas 7. Grease and line a 32 × 23cm/13 × 9in Swiss roll tin with baking parchment.

2. Drain the spinach well by pressing against a sieve to remove excess water, and then pat dry using kitchen paper. Transfer to a bowl and mix with the egg yolks, nutmeg and seasoning.

3. In another bowl, whisk the egg whites until very frothy but not too stiff, and fold into the spinach mixture. Spread into the prepared tin and smooth the top. Bake for 12-15 minutes until firm and golden.

4. Meanwhile, blend the pepper and passata together in a food processor or blender until smooth, season and set aside. Beat the soft cheese to soften and stir in the fromage frais, chives, Parmesan cheese and seasoning.

5. Turn the spinach base on to a sheet of baking parchment and peel away the lining paper. Spread the cheese and chive mixture over the spinach to cover it completely.

6. Holding the end of the paper, carefully roll up the spinach base like a Swiss roll. Press gently to seal the edge.

7. Transfer the pepper and tomato mixture to a small saucepan and heat through. Slice the roulade thinly and serve with the sauce spooned over.

mushrooms à la greque

A simple, yet tasty starter making the most of the meaty texture of mushrooms. Experiment with different varieties of mushrooms as there are so many to choose from nowadays. Serve this dish simply with a few salad leaves.

Serves: 4
Preparation time: approximately
10 minutes plus cooling and chilling
Cooking time: approximately
5 minutes

227g/8oz baby button mushrooms
227g/8oz open cup mushrooms
284ml/½pt vegetable stock
2 bay leaves
397g/14oz can chopped tomatoes with garlic
4 tbsp dry white wine
Salt and freshly ground black pepper
4 tbsp freshly chopped parsley
28g/1oz pitted black olives in brine, drained and roughly chopped

1. Wipe the mushrooms. Place the baby button mushrooms in a saucepan. Thickly slice the open cup mushrooms and add to the saucepan along with the stock and bay leaves. Bring to the boil, cover and simmer for 5 minutes until just tender. Remove from the heat and allow to cool.

2. Drain the mushrooms and discard the bay leaves. Carefully mix in the tomatoes, wine and seasoning. Cover and chill for at least an hour.

3. To serve, sprinkle each portion with chopped parsley and a few chopped olives.

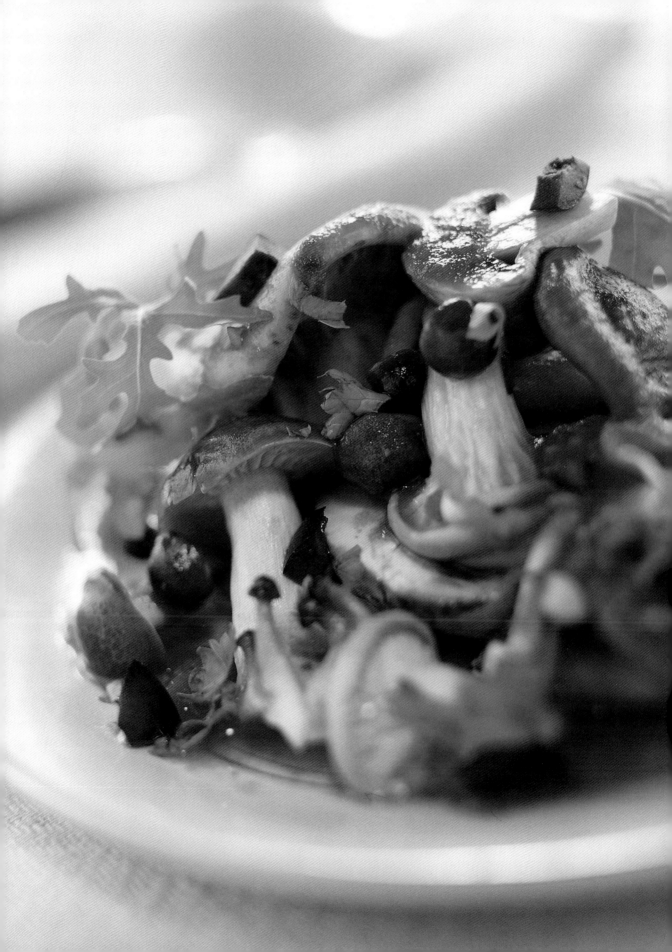

gingered vegetable filo parcels

Impressive, crisp parcels of filo pastry filled with shredded Oriental-style vegetables make an excellent and stylish way to start a special meal. You can try other vegetable combinations such as cauliflower, potato and peas flavoured with mild curry spices.

Serves: 4

Preparation time: approximately 20 minutes

Cooking time: approximately 20 minutes

1 large carrot
170g/6oz piece celeriac
2.5cm/1in piece root ginger
2 spring onions
1 tsp sesame oil
2 tsp dark soy sauce
2 x 28g/1oz large sheets frozen filo pastry, thawed
1 medium egg, beaten
2 level tsp sesame seeds

1. Preheat the oven to 200°C/400°F/Gas 6. Peel the carrot and celeriac. Coarsely grate or cut into fine shreds, and place in a bowl. Peel and finely grate the ginger and mix into the vegetables.

2. Trim and finely chop the white and green parts of the spring onions and mix into the vegetables along with the sesame oil and soy sauce. Set aside.

3. Lay the pastry sheets on top of each other and cut into quarters. Brush four pieces of filo pastry with egg and lay another piece on top at a different angle to form a cross shape. Brush with more egg.

4. Pile some vegetables in the centre of each and bring up the pastry edges, scrunching them together at the top to form 'purses'.

5. Transfer to a baking sheet lined with baking parchment and brush with more egg. Sprinkle lightly with sesame seeds and bake for 15-20 minutes until golden and cooked through. Best served hot.

Cook's Note

If celeriac is unavailable, then replace with a stick of celery. Simply trim and finely chop.

chicken gumbo

This soup comes from Louisiana in the southern states of America. It uses the vegetable okra, which when cut exudes a sticky white paste that thickens soups and stews. If okra is unavailable, you can use courgettes instead.

Serves: 4
Preparation time: approximately
15 minutes
Cooking time: approximately
30 minutes

1 large onion
1 garlic clove
1 stick celery
284ml/½pt chicken stock
made with Bovril
1 large green pepper
227g/8oz okra
2 x 397g/14oz cans chopped
tomatoes
85g/3oz garlic sausage
340g/12oz lean cooked
skinless, boneless chicken
Salt and freshly ground
black pepper
2 tbsp freshly chopped
parsley

1. Peel and finely chop the onion and garlic. Trim and chop the celery. Place in a large saucepan and pour over half the stock. Bring to the boil, cover and simmer for 5 minutes.

2. Meanwhile, halve and de-seed the pepper. Cut into small pieces. Trim the okra and slice into 1cm/½in pieces. Stir into the saucepan along with the remaining stock and chopped tomatoes. Bring to the boil, cover and simmer for 15 minutes.

3. Chop the sausage into small pieces and slice the chicken into bite-sized chunks.

4. Stir the sausage and chicken into the saucepan and season well. Bring back to the boil and simmer, uncovered, for 5 minutes until thoroughly heated through.

5. Ladle into warmed soup bowls and serve sprinkled with chopped parsley.

peperonata filo tarts

The wafer-thin layers of pastry in these tarts make them perfect for Syn watching. The tasty filling of peppers and onion is topped with a cheesy layer, which sets on baking. They are best served straight from the oven.

Serves: 4
Preparation time: approximately
15 minutes
Cooking time: approximately
50 minutes

1 small red pepper
1 small red onion
1 large beefsteak tomato
Salt and freshly ground
black pepper
Fry Light
2 x 28g/1oz large sheets
frozen filo pastry, thawed
1 medium egg, beaten
4 tbsp very low-fat fromage
frais
2 level tbsp freshly grated
Parmesan cheese
1 tsp dried oregano

1. Preheat the oven to 200°C/400°F/Gas 6. Halve and de-seed the pepper and cut in half again. Peel the onion and cut into quarters. Remove the stalk from the tomato and cut in half.

2. Arrange the vegetables on a non-stick baking sheet or small shallow roasting tin. Season well and spray lightly with Fry Light. Bake in the oven for 25-30 minutes until tender.

3. Meanwhile, lay the sheets of pastry on top of each other and cut into six equal pieces. Lay one piece of pastry in the base of four 10cm/4in square non-stick Yorkshire pudding tins. Brush with a little egg and lay another piece on top at a different angle. Brush again and top with the remaining pastry. Push in the edges slightly to create a case.

4. Mix the remaining egg with the fromage frais, Parmesan cheese and seasoning.

5. Once the vegetables are cooked, chop them roughly and mix them together. Pile into the pastry cases and top with the cheese mixture. Sprinkle with oregano and bake in the oven for 15-20 minutes until golden and set. Best served warm.

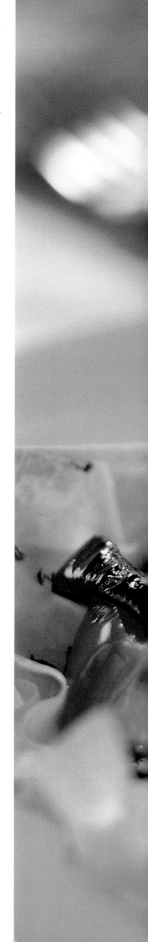

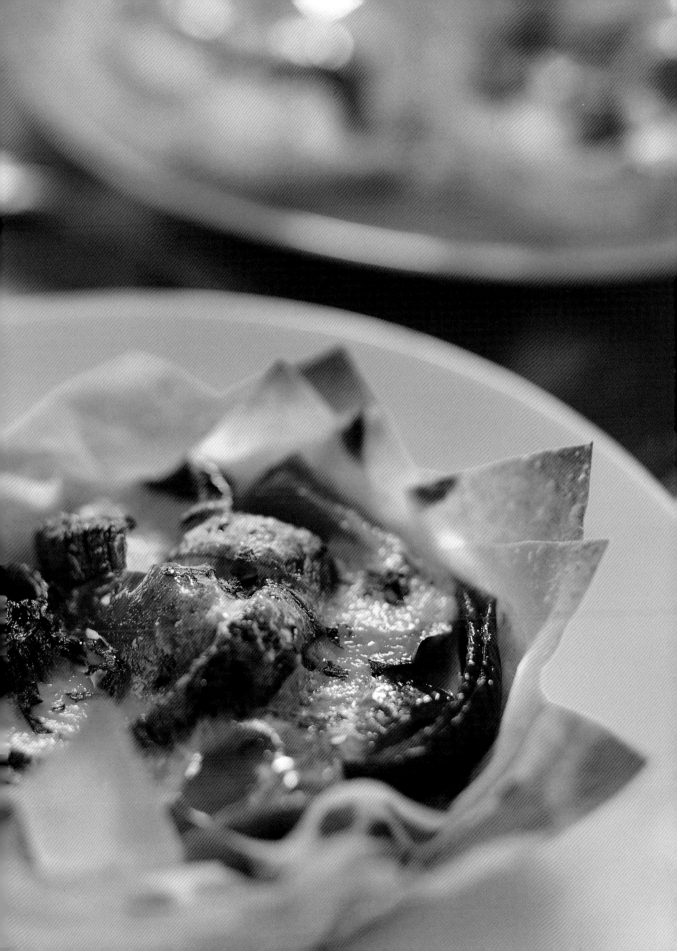

chinese chicken and mushroom soup

This clear soup makes an excellent choice to start a heavier meal. It is a good way to use up leftover cooked meat – turkey or pork would also work well. Remember that soy sauce is very salty so you won't need any more seasoning.

Serves: 4
Preparation time: approximately
15 minutes
Cooking time: approximately
8 minutes

170g/6oz baby corn
1 bunch spring onions
1cm/½in piece root ginger
113g/4oz small shiitake or
button mushrooms
340g/12oz lean cooked
skinless, boneless chicken
2 tbsp dark soy sauce
2 tbsp dry sherry
2 level tsp light brown sugar
1.2 litres/2pt chicken stock
made with Bovril

1. Trim the baby corn and slice in half lengthwise. Trim the spring onions, reserving two for garnish, chop the remaining. Peel and grate the ginger. Wipe and slice the mushrooms.

2. Slice the chicken into thin shreds and place in a bowl. Stir in the spring onions, ginger, mushrooms, soy sauce, sherry and sugar. Mix well and set aside.

3. Pour the stock into a large saucepan and bring to the boil. Add the baby corn and simmer for 1 minute. Stir in the chicken mixture, bring back to the boil and simmer for 5 minutes until thoroughly heated through and tender.

4. Meanwhile, finely shred or chop the reserved spring onions. To serve, ladle the soup into warmed soup bowls and sprinkle with spring onions.

classic leek and potato soup

Traditionally, this soup has butter and thick cream added to it, but our version is much lighter and allows the subtle flavour of the vegetables to come through. This is the perfect choice for those who prefer a less strongly flavoured soup.

Serves: 4
Preparation time: approximately
10 minutes
Cooking time: approximately
35 minutes

1 large onion
2 bay leaves
1.2 litres/2pt chicken stock
made with Bovril
681g/1½lb potatoes
1 large leek
Salt and freshly ground
black pepper
142g/5oz very low-fat
natural fromage frais
2 tbsp freshly chopped
chives

1. Peel and finely chop the onion. Place in a large saucepan along with the bay leaves and 142ml/¼pt of the stock. Bring to the boil, cover and simmer for 5 minutes.

2. Meanwhile, peel and finely dice the potatoes. Trim the leek and slice lengthwise. Rinse under cold water to remove any trapped earth. Shake well to remove excess water and then shred.

3. Add the potato and all but a few shreds of the leek. Pour in the remaining stock and season well. Bring to the boil, cover and simmer for 25 minutes until tender.

4. Discard the bay leaves and transfer the mixture to a food processor or blender. Blend until smooth and return to the saucepan.

5. Blend in the fromage frais and reheat gently without boiling. Adjust the seasoning if necessary. Ladle into warmed soup bowls, sprinkle with black pepper, reserved shredded leek and chopped chives.

italian-style bacon soup with pesto

Pesto sauce is full of Syns, but this version although lighter, still has all the flavour and is delicious spooned on to a hot, chunky soup such as this. As the pesto starts to melt, it runs into the soup and adds a more intense flavour.

Serves: 4
Preparation time: approximately
15 minutes
Cooking time: approximately
25 minutes

113g/4oz lean unsmoked
rindless back bacon
1 large onion
1 large carrot
2 sticks celery
284ml/½pt vegetable stock
1 medium red pepper
1 tsp dried oregano
2 x 397g/14oz can chopped
tomatoes with garlic
Salt and freshly ground
black pepper
4 tbsp very low-fat fromage
frais
2 level tbsp freshly grated
Parmesan cheese
1 garlic clove (optional)
A small bunch fresh basil
Small basil leaves to garnish

1. Remove any excess fat from the bacon and then finely chop. Place in a large non-stick saucepan. Peel and finely chop the onion and add to the saucepan. Heat gently until the bacon juices run, and then stir fry for 2-3 minutes.

2. Peel and finely chop the carrot. Trim and chop the celery. Stir into the bacon and pour over half the stock. Bring to the boil, cover and simmer for 5 minutes.

3. Halve and de-seed the pepper, then cut into small pieces. Add to the saucepan along with the oregano, tomatoes, remaining stock and seasoning. Bring to the boil, and simmer for 15 minutes until thick and tender.

4. Meanwhile, prepare the pesto. Mix the fromage frais and Parmesan cheese together. Peel and crush the garlic, if using, and stir into the mixture along with some seasoning. Chop the basil finely and add to the mixture. Cover and chill until required.

5. To serve, ladle the soup into warmed soup bowls. Top each with a spoonful of pesto, sprinkle over black pepper and a few basil leaves.

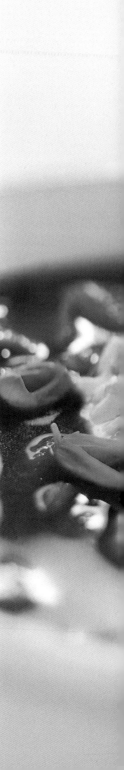

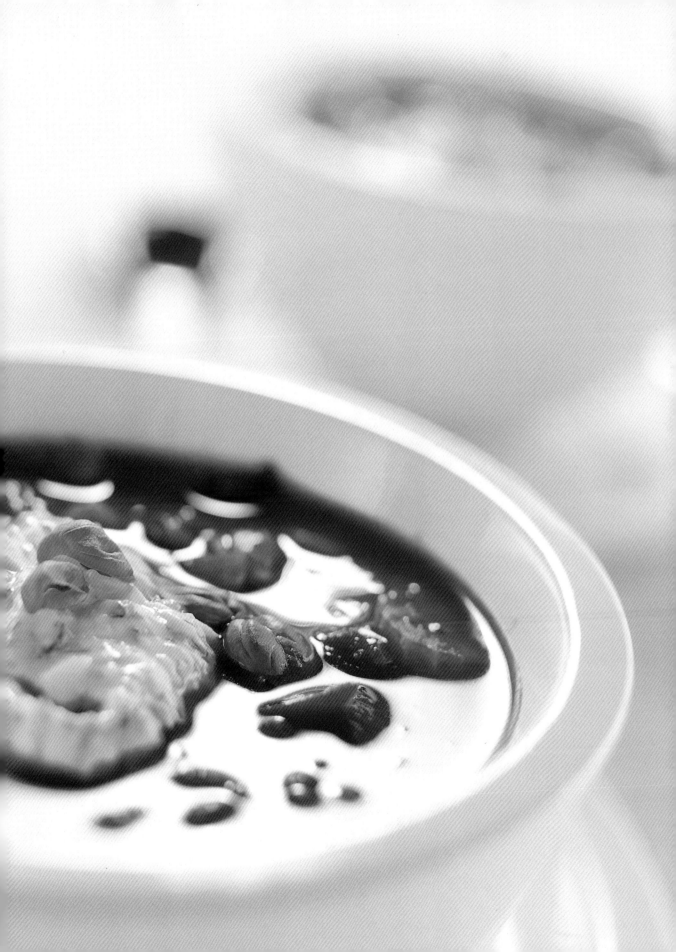

french-style fish soup

A popular dish all along the shores of the Mediterranean; French fish soup is more of a stew than a soup, but is light enough to serve as a starter. You can use one type of fish or shellfish if you prefer.

Serves: 4
Preparation time: approximately
15 minutes
Cooking time: approximately
25 minutes

1 large red onion
2 garlic cloves
1 tbsp lemon juice
A few sprigs fresh thyme or
½ tsp dried
A few sprigs fresh rosemary
or ½ tsp dried
142ml/¼pt dry white wine
2 x 397g/14oz cans chopped
tomatoes
284ml/½pt fish stock
567g/1lb 4oz skinless firm
white fish fillets such as cod,
haddock or plaice
227g/8oz peeled large
prawns, thawed if frozen
227g/8oz cooked shelled
mussels, thawed if frozen
Salt and freshly ground
black pepper
Fresh thyme and rosemary
to garnish

1. Peel and finely chop the onion and garlic. Place in a large saucepan along with the lemon juice, herbs and wine. Bring to the boil, cover and simmer for 5 minutes.

2. Stir in the tomatoes and stock, bring to the boil and simmer for a further 10 minutes. Meanwhile, wash and pat dry the white fish, prawns and mussels. Cut the fish into 2.5cm/1in cubes.

3. Stir the cubed fish into the saucepan, mix well and simmer, covered, for 5 minutes until the fish is opaque. Stir in the prawns, mussels and plenty of seasoning, and continue to simmer, covered, for a further 2-3 minutes until tender and cooked through.

4. Ladle into warmed soup bowls, sprinkle with black pepper, garnish and serve with wedges of lemon to squeeze over.

gazpacho with prawns

Gazpacho with prawns is perfect for a summer meal. If you've never tried a cold soup before then this is the one for you. Because the vegetables are raw, you get all their flavour and colour – it's really like a salad juice in a bowl!

Serves: 4
Preparation time: approximately
25 minutes plus chilling

4 large beefsteak tomatoes
I medium red onion
I garlic clove
½ cucumber
2 sticks celery
I large red pepper
Juice of I large lemon
284ml/½pt passata
2 tbsp white wine vinegar
1-2 tsp granulated artificial
sweetener
Salt and freshly ground
black pepper
A few ice cubes
340g/12oz peeled prawns,
thawed if frozen
I tbsp freshly chopped
chives

1. Wash, pat dry and remove the stalk from the tomatoes. Roughly chop and place in a food processor or blender. Peel and roughly chop the onion, garlic and cucumber and add to the tomatoes.

2. Wash, pat dry, trim and roughly chop the celery. Wash, pat dry and halve the pepper. De-seed and roughly chop. Place both vegetables in the food processor along with the lemon juice and blend until well processed and smooth – you may find it easier to do this in two batches.

3. Place a large sieve over a basin and push the puréed vegetables through to form a smooth liquid. Stir in the passata and vinegar, and add sufficient sweetener and seasoning to taste. Cover and chill for 1 hour.

4. To serve, arrange a few ice cubes in four serving bowls and spoon over the chilled soup. Sprinkle with prawns, black pepper and a few chives.

hearty bean and vegetable soup

Using canned pulses and beans is great for labour saving. Keep them in the cupboard as a good standby for when you want to make a vegetable stew or soup more substantial. They're an excellent source of dietary fibre as well.

Serves: 4
Preparation time: approximately
10 minutes
Cooking time: approximately
30 minutes

1 medium onion
1 garlic clove
1 tsp dried oregano
284ml/½pt vegetable stock
1 large green pepper
420g/15oz can mixed pulses,
drained and rinsed
568ml/1pt passata
1 large courgette
326g/11oz can sweetcorn
kernels in water, drained
Salt and freshly ground
black pepper
Fresh oregano leaves

1. Peel and finely chop the onion and garlic. Place in a large saucepan along with the oregano and half the stock. Bring to the boil, cover and simmer for 5 minutes.

2. Meanwhile, halve and de-seed the pepper. Cut into small chunks. Stir the pepper, pulses and passata into the onion along with the remaining stock. Bring to the boil, cover and simmer for 10 minutes.

3. Trim and dice the courgette into small chunks and stir into the soup along with the sweetcorn. Simmer for a further 10 minutes. Taste and season.

4. Ladle into warmed soup bowls, garnish with fresh oregano leaves and serve.

middle eastern spiced lentil broth

A warming combination of sweet spices makes this an interesting and tasty choice for a supper dish. It is very substantial and is excellent served with a chopped cucumber and coriander salad mixed with low-fat yogurt.

Serves: 4
Preparation time: approximately
10 minutes
Cooking time: approximately
1 hour 10 minutes

1 large onion
1 tsp ground cinnamon
1 tsp ground cumin
1 tsp ground coriander
852ml/1½pt chicken stock
made with Bovril
113g/4oz raw/dried
red lentils
397g/14oz can chopped
tomatoes with garlic
Salt and freshly ground
black pepper
4 baby aubergines
2 tbsp freshly chopped
coriander

1. Peel and finely chop the onion. Place in a large saucepan with the spices and 142ml/¼pt of the vegetable stock. Bring to the boil, cover and simmer for 5 minutes.

2. Stir in the lentils with the remaining stock and chopped tomatoes. Season well, bring to the boil, cover and simmer gently for 45 minutes – keep the heat low and stir occasionally to prevent the soup sticking on the bottom of the saucepan.

3. Trim and finely dice the aubergines and stir into the soup. Continue to simmer for a further 15 minutes until tender and very thick.

4. Adjust the seasoning if necessary. Ladle into warmed soup bowls and sprinkle with chopped coriander to serve.

Cook's Note
If preferred, replace the baby aubergine with a small, standard aubergine.

mixed root vegetable soup

A colourful combination of vegetables makes a hearty supper. Make sure you choose beetroot cooked in natural juice and not in vinegar, as this will spoil the flavour of the finished dish.

Serves: 4
Preparation time: approximately
15 minutes
Cooking time: approximately
40 minutes

1 large onion
1 stick celery
2 bay leaves
1.2 litres/2pt vegetable stock
1 large potato
2 large carrots
250g/8oz pack cooked
beetroot in natural juice
Salt and freshly ground
black pepper
4 tbsp very low-fat natural
fromage frais
1 tbsp freshly chopped
parsley

1. Peel and finely chop the onion. Trim and finely chop the celery. Place in a large saucepan with the bay leaves and pour in 142ml/¼pt of the stock. Bring to the boil, cover and simmer for 5 minutes until tender.

2. Meanwhile, peel and dice the potato into small chunks. Peel and finely chop the carrots. Add to the onion and celery, and pour in the remaining stock. Bring to the boil, cover and simmer for 25 minutes until tender. Drain and finely dice the beetroot into small chunks and add to the saucepan. Simmer for a further 5 minutes. Discard the bay leaves.

3. Transfer to a blender or food processor and process for a few seconds until smooth – you may find it easier to do this in two batches. Taste and season.

4. Reheat the soup if necessary. Ladle into warmed soup bowls and top each with some fromage frais, more black pepper and a little chopped parsley.

roast mediterranean vegetable soup

The selection of vegetables in this soup has become a classic in our diet, but the addition of squash gives a slightly buttery, earthy flavour, and an excellent golden colour. You can roast the vegetables the day before if you prefer.

Serves: 4
Preparation time: approximately
15 minutes
Cooking time: approximately
35 minutes

1 small butternut squash
1 medium red pepper
1 medium yellow pepper
1 large red onion
2 large beefsteak tomatoes
2 garlic cloves
Juice of 1 lemon
A few sprigs fresh rosemary
Salt and freshly ground
black pepper
Fry Light
1.2 litres/2pt chicken stock
made with Bovril
Rosemary to garnish

1. Preheat the oven to 200°C/400°F/Gas 6. Halve the squash and scoop out the seeds. Cut each half into four equal pieces. Halve and de-seed the peppers, and cut each half into four pieces.

2. Peel the onion and cut into thick wedges. Remove the stalks from the tomatoes and cut in half. Arrange all the vegetables on a large, non-stick baking sheet or shallow roasting tin.

3. Peel the garlic and slice thinly. Sprinkle over the vegetables along with the lemon juice. Scatter the rosemary on top and season well. Spray lightly with Fry Light and bake in the oven for 30 minutes or until tender.

4. Discard the rosemary. Scoop out the flesh from the squash and place in a food processor or blender. Reserving a piece of each pepper and some onion for garnish, add all the other vegetables and 426ml/¾pt stock, and process for a few seconds until smooth.

5. Transfer to a large saucepan and stir in the remaining stock. Heat through for 4-5 minutes until piping hot.

6. Adjust the seasoning if necessary and ladle into warmed soup bowls. Slice the reserved peppers and onion and place on top along with fresh rosemary to garnish.

prawn and melon cocktail

This is a variation of the classic starter of the Sixties and Seventies. It has been brought right up to date and can look stunning when piled up on serving plates. Your guests will think you've spent ages preparing this dish, but it is very simple, and very tasty.

Serves: 4

Preparation and cooking time: approximately 25 minutes

8 thin slices lean Parma ham
1 head of radicchio lettuce
½ orange-fleshed melon such as charantais
½ green-fleshed melon such as galia
340g/12oz peeled prawns, thawed if frozen
1 level tbsp low-calorie mayonnaise
1 tbsp very low-fat natural fromage frais
½ tsp mild curry powder
2 level tsp spicy mango chutney
Salt and freshly ground black pepper
2 tbsp freshly chopped coriander

1. Preheat the grill to a hot setting. Trim away any excess fat from the ham and lay the slices side by side on the grill rack. Cook under the grill for about a minutes, turning, until wrinkled and crispy. Drain and set aside.

2. Trim away the outside leaves from the lettuce. Wash and shake dry, then break up the leaves and arrange on four serving plates.

3. Halve the melons and scoop out the seeds. Trim away the skin and cut the melons into bite-sized pieces and place on top of the lettuce. Top with the prawns.

4. Mix together the mayonnaise, fromage frais, curry powder, chutney and seasoning and spoon on top of the prawns. Arrange the ham on top either whole or broken up and sprinkle with chopped coriander before serving.

Cook's Note
Radicchio is a slightly bitter-tasting, deep reddish-pink leaf which looks stunning in salads. If preferred, you can use a selection of small lettuce leaves or Little Gem lettuce.

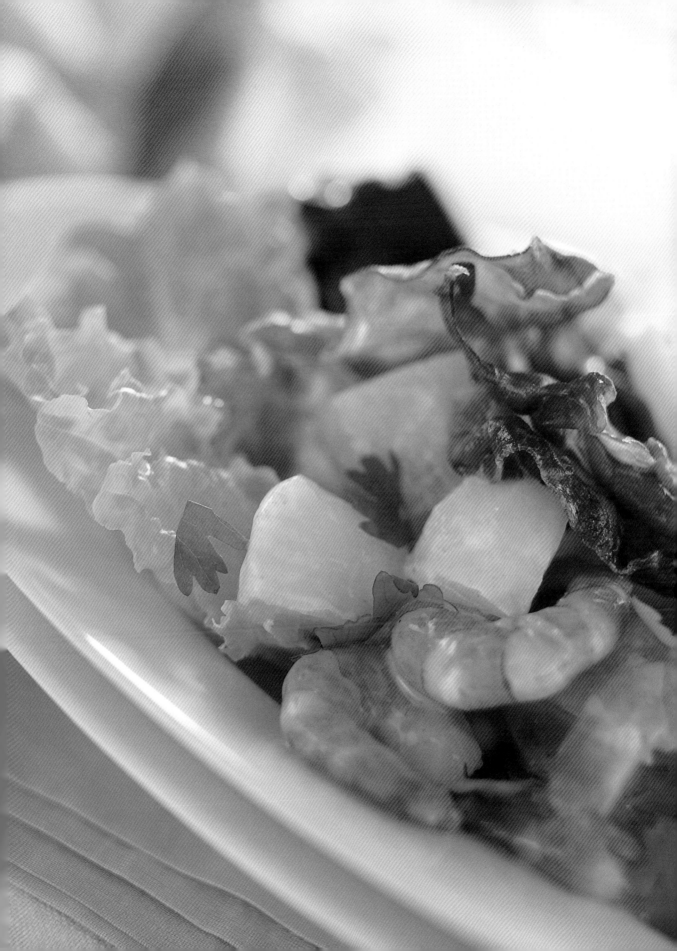

insalata di mare

An Italian-style seafood salad. You can buy ready-cooked and prepared selections of seafood, which you could use instead, and which would be even easier to use. Chilling the seafood in the dressing allows the flavours to develop and makes for a more flavoursome dish.

Serves: 4
Preparation time: approximately
10 minutes plus chilling

227g/8oz peeled prawns, thawed if frozen
113g/4oz cooked, shelled mussels
113g/4oz cooked squid rings
170g/6oz can white crab meat, drained
Juice and finely grated rind of 1 lemon
2 tbsp fat-free vinaigrette salad dressing
2 tbsp freshly chopped parsley
Salt and freshly ground pepper
4 large whole prawns
8 green or New Zealand mussels (optional)
Lemon zest and parsley sprigs to garnish

1. Wash and pat dry the prawns, mussels and squid and place in a bowl. Flake the crab meat and mix into the fishes along with the lemon juice, salad dressing, chopped parsley and seasoning. Cover and chill for 30 minutes.

2. To serve, pile on to four serving plates and serve each portion with a whole prawn and two green mussels, if using. Garnish and serve with extra lemon if liked.

smoked fish pâté

Very easy to prepare, this pâté also makes a good filling for sandwiches. It can easily be packed in a box for a picnic or packed lunch as it is quite firm once chilled. If you haven't got a food processor, then mash the fish with a fork for a chunkier result.

Serves: 4
Preparation time: approximately
20 minutes plus chilling

397g/14oz red or pink salmon canned in brine, drained
113g/4oz smoked mackerel fillet
113g/4oz quark skimmed milk soft cheese
Juice of 1 small lemon
Salt and freshly ground black pepper
57g/2oz smoked salmon
2 tbsp freshly chopped parsley

1. Flake the salmon away from the skin and bones and place in a mixing bowl. Skin and flake the mackerel and mix into the salmon.

2. Mix the cheese and lemon juice into the fishes until well combined. Taste and season if necessary.

3. Shred or finely chop the smoked salmon and mix into the pâté. If you want a smoother pâté, then blend in the food processor for a few seconds. Cover and chill for 30 minutes.

4. Serve scooped on to serving plates, sprinkled with chopped parsley. Accompany with wedges of lemon to squeeze over, and mixed salad or sticks of raw vegetables.

terrine of chicken

This meaty loaf is a classic starter. Although it takes a while to prepare and cook, the flavour is very intense and well worth the effort. Wrap and chill for up to five days, or slice and freeze in individual portions for easy serving.

Serves: 4-6
Preparation time: approximately
25 minutes plus cooling and chilling
Cooking time: approximately
1 hour 25 minutes

4 rashers lean rindless,
unsmoked back bacon
113g/4oz button
mushrooms
1 garlic clove
142ml/¼pt vegetable stock
454g/1lb chicken livers,
thawed if frozen
3 tbsp dry red wine
1 tsp dried thyme
1 tbsp brandy
1 medium red pepper
1 medium yellow pepper
227g/8oz skinless boneless
chicken breasts
1 medium egg, beaten
Salt and freshly ground
black pepper

1. Preheat the oven to 180°C/350°F/Gas 4. Remove all visible fat from the bacon and lay the bacon rashers overlapping in the base of a 908g/2lb non-stick loaf tin, and chill until required.

2. Wipe and slice the mushrooms. Peel and finely chop the garlic. Place both in a saucepan along with the stock. Bring to the boil, cover and simmer for 5 minutes.

3. Meanwhile, mince the chicken livers. Add to the saucepan along with the wine, thyme and brandy. Simmer gently, stirring, for 5 minutes. Remove from the heat and allow to cool.

4. Halve and de-seed the peppers. Slice thinly lengthwise. Slice the chicken into thin strips. Cover and chill until required.

5. To assemble the terrine, mix the egg and plenty of seasoning into the chicken liver mixture and spoon one-third into the base of the prepared tin. Cover with a single layer of pepper strips and half the chicken strips. Spoon over half the remaining mixture and arrange the remaining pepper and chicken over the top. Spread over the remaining mixture and cover with foil.

6. Stand the loaf tin in a roasting tin and pour sufficient boiling water into the tin to come half way up the sides of the tin. Bake in the oven for 1 hour 10 minutes or until set and the juices run clear when a skewer is inserted into the middle. Remove from the water and carefully drain away the cooking juices from the terrine. Allow to cool, then chill for at least 2 hours.

7. Loosen the terrine from the tin by running a pallet knife around the edge and then turn out. Serve sliced with assorted salad leaves and cherry tomatoes.

waldorf stuffed pear
with parma ham

Choose ripe pears for this dish as it will make all the difference to the final taste. Ripen pears on the windowsill in a brown paper bag for one or two days before you make this starter to ensure they really are nice and juicy.

Serves: 4
Preparation time: approximately
20 minutes

1 eating apple
2 tbsp lemon juice
28g/1oz Stilton cheese
113g/4oz quark skimmed
milk soft cheese
1 tbsp freshly chopped
parsley
Salt and freshly ground
black pepper
4 ripe pears
1 bunch watercress
2 walnut halves
8 thin slices lean Parma
ham

1. Peel, core and grate the apple, and mix with half the lemon juice. Place in a mixing bowl. Crumble in the Stilton cheese and add the quark, parsley and seasoning. Mix well until combined. Set aside.

2. Wash and pat dry the pears. Halve and scoop out the core, leaving the stalk intact. Brush all over with the remaining lemon juice, and pile the cheese mixture on top of each.

3. Wash and shake dry the watercress and divide between four serving plates. Arrange the pear halves on top.

4. Lightly crush the walnuts and sprinkle over. Trim the ham and roll up tightly. Place on top of each portion to serve.

chicken tikka

Chicken tikka is now one of Britain's favourite meals, and there's no reason why slimmers should miss out on it! This quick and easy version tastes fantastic and is ideal served as a starter. The longer you let the chicken marinate in the spicy yogurt, the better the flavour. But if time is short, the 30 minutes estimated here is fine.

Serves: 4
Preparation and cooking time:
approximately 30 minutes plus
chilling

4 boneless, skinless chicken breasts
Salt and freshly ground black pepper
6 tbsp very low-fat natural yogurt
1 level tbsp tomato purée
1 tbsp medium curry powder
1 tbsp lemon juice
2 tbsp freshly chopped coriander

1. Wash and pat dry the chicken breasts. Using a small sharp knife, slice the breasts three or four times diagonally without cutting right the way through. Season both sides with salt and freshly ground black pepper and place in a shallow dish.

2. Mix the remaining ingredients together and spoon over the chicken, making sure the chicken is completely covered. Cover and chill for at least 30 minutes.

3. Preheat the grill to medium/hot. Line the grill tray with foil and arrange the chicken breasts in the tray. Cook the chicken for 8-10 minutes on each side or until tender and cooked through.

4. Drain the chicken and serve with raita (diced cucumber and yogurt) and a tomato, onion and mixed green leaf salad.

crispy potato skins

Potatoes are a real comfort food and this recipe is no exception. It makes a delicious starter or snack served with a crisp salad.

Serves:4
Preparation and cooking time:
approximately 1 hour

**4 x 227g/8oz baking
potatoes
Salt**

1. Scrub the potatoes and bake in a preheated oven at 200°C/400°F/Gas 6 for about 1 hour, until tender.

2. Cut the potatoes in half lengthwise, scoop out most of the flesh, leaving a thin layer of potato around the inside of each shell and cut in half again making 16 quarters.

3. Season the shells lightly with salt and spoon in the filling of your choice.

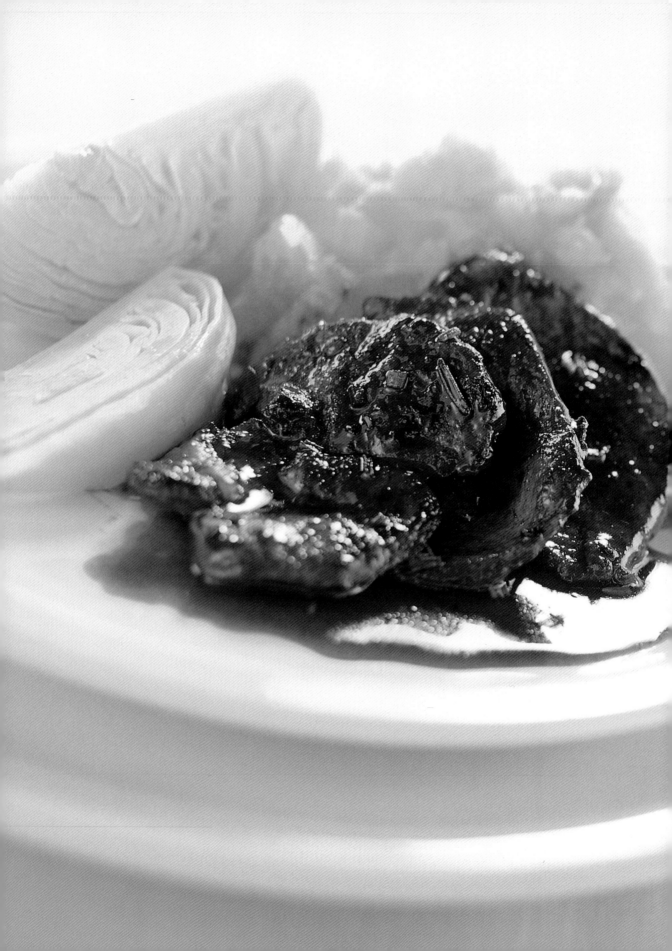

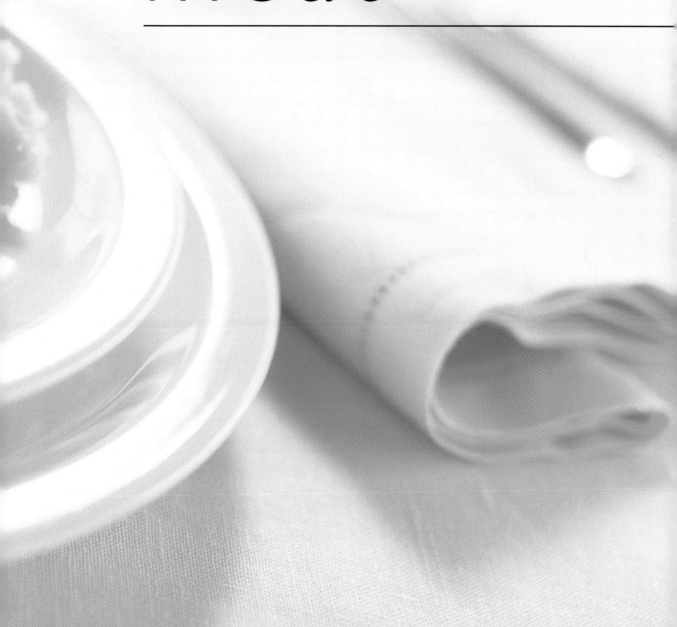

main courses:
meat

meatloaf with spinach and pepper stuffing

Meatloaf is a classic family favourite. This particular version has a middle layer of spinach and peppers and is served with a tasty tomato sauce quickly made in 5 minutes.

Serves: 4
Preparation time: approximately
20 minutes plus standing
Cooking time: approximately
1 hour

1 small onion
681g/1½lb extra lean minced beef
4 tbsp freshly chopped parsley
Salt and freshly ground black pepper
1 medium egg yolk
1 small red pepper
113g/4oz frozen chopped spinach, drained
284ml/½pt passata
142ml/¼pt dry white wine
½ tsp dried onion powder
½ tsp dried thyme

1. Preheat the oven to 190°C/375°F/Gas 5. Grease and line a 908g/2lb loaf tin with baking parchment. Peel and finely chop the onion and place in a mixing bowl with the minced beef, 2 tbsp parsley, seasoning and the egg yolk. Mix until well combined.

2. Halve and de-seed the pepper and cut into thin strips. Press the spinach against the side of a colander or sieve to make sure it is thoroughly drained.

3. Divide the beef mixture in half and press half into the bottom of the tin. Make an indent down the centre of the beef and lay the spinach and peppers down its length. Top with remaining beef, packing it down well.

4. Cover the top of the tin with a layer of baking parchment and then foil. Bake for about 1 hour or until tender and cooked through, and the juices run clear when a skewer is inserted into the middle. Stand for 10 minutes, then drain away any juices.

5. While the loaf is standing, pour the passata, wine, onion powder, thyme and seasoning into a small saucepan. Bring to the boil and simmer for 5 minutes.

6. Carefully remove the loaf from the tin and sprinkle with the remaining parsley. Serve in slices with the tomato and wine sauce to accompany.

pizzaiola steak

This dish is ideal served when entertaining and is extremely easy to cook. The tomato-based sauce makes a change from the standard sauces served with steaks.

Serves: 4
Preparation and cooking time:
approximately 30 minutes

681g/1½lb fresh plum tomatoes
1 medium onion
1 garlic clove
4 tbsp vegetable stock
1 tbsp freshly chopped marjoram or 1 tsp dried
1 level tbsp tomato purée
1 tsp granulated artificial sweetener
Salt and freshly ground black pepper
4 x 170g/6oz sirloin or rump steaks
1 tsp olive oil
2 tbsp freshly chopped parsley

1. Prick the tomatoes with a fork and stand them in a large heatproof bowl covered in boiling water for 2 minutes until the skin comes away. Drain and peel the tomatoes. Halve and de-seed, and then chop the flesh and set aside.

2. Peel and finely chop the onion and garlic. Place in a saucepan with the stock. Bring to the boil and simmer for 4-5 minutes until tender. Stir in the tomatoes, marjoram, tomato purée, sweetener and seasoning. Add 2 tbsp water, bring to the boil and simmer gently for 10 minutes, stirring occasionally.

3. Meanwhile, trim the steaks and remove any visible fat. Brush a ridged or non-stick frying pan with the oil and heat until hot. Add the steaks, pressing on the pan, and cook for 4-5 minutes on each side, lowering the heat after 1 minute, until cooked to your liking.

4. Stir the parsley into the tomato sauce. Drain the steaks and serve with the tomato sauce spooned over.

teriyaki beef
and orange skewers

Another really quick and easy dish, which is also delicious barbecued. Serve the skewers of beef and orange with a crisp green salad.

Serves: 4
Preparation and cooking time:
30 minutes

454g/1lb lean beef steak
2 medium oranges
1 clove garlic
4 tbsp dark soy sauce
1 tbsp dry sherry
1 level tbsp clear honey
1 tsp sesame oil
2 spring onions

1. Soak eight bamboo skewers in warm water. Meanwhile, trim any visible fat from the steak, slice into long thin strips and place in a shallow dish.

2. Cut the top and bottom off each orange and slice off the skin and pith. Holding the orange over the beef dish, cut out each portion of flesh from the orange segments, allowing juice and segments to fall in the dish. Peel and crush the garlic and mix into the beef with soy sauce, sherry, honey and oil. Thread the beef in 'S' shapes down each skewer with a few orange segments. Reserve the juices.

3. Cover the ends of the skewers with foil and cook under a medium grill for 3-4 minutes each side, brushing with reserved juices to prevent drying. Trim and shred the spring onions and sprinkle over the skewers for the last minute of grilling.

4. Strain remaining juices into a small pan, bring to the boil and simmer for 1-2 minutes until syrupy. Serve two skewers per portion drizzled with the syrup.

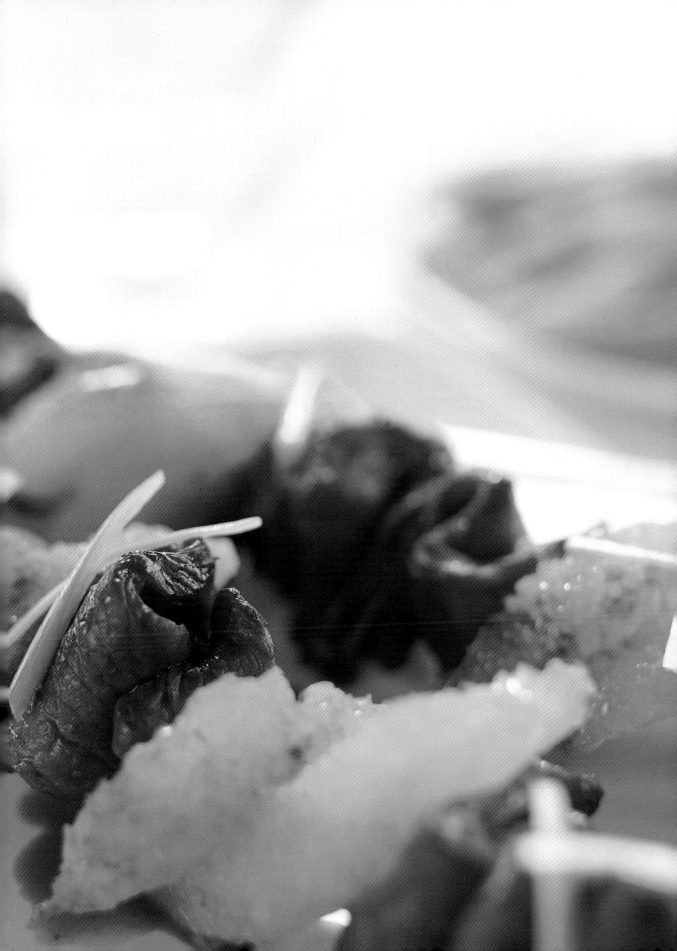

chicken and pumpkin casserole

The ultimate in comfort food, this flavoursome and chunky Italian-style casserole is the perfect way to spiece up autumn days. If pumpkin is not in season, use any type of squash.

Serves: 4
Preparation and cooking time:
approximately 1 hour

4 x 227g/8oz part-boned
chicken breasts, skinned
Salt and freshly ground
black pepper
2 tsp dried basil
1 tsp olive oil
1 garlic clove
1 medium red onion
454g/1lb pumpkin
2 x 397g/14oz cans chopped
tomatoes
1 lemon
2 bay leaves
4 small courgettes
1 medium yellow pepper
2 tsp granulated artificial
sweetener
28g/1oz pitted black olives,
halved
A few leaves fresh basil,
shredded

1. Wash the chicken breasts and pat dry with kitchen paper. Rub with seasoning and dried basil. Brush a ridged non-stick frying pan with oil and heat until hot. Press the chicken into the pan for 1 minute each side, over a high heat, to seal – do two at a time if the pan is small. Drain on kitchen paper and set aside.

2. Peel and finely chop the garlic, peel and slice the onion. Place in a large saucepan with a tightly fitting lid. Using a small sharp knife, slice off the hard skin from the pumpkin, and then scoop out and discard the seeds. Slice into wedges and then into 2.5cm/1in chunks. Place in the saucepan.

3. Pour in the chopped tomatoes and mix well. Push the chicken breasts into the mixture. Using a vegetable peeler, pare off a few strips of lemon rind into the saucepan and add the bay leaves. Squeeze the lemon juice and pour it into the saucepan. Bring to the boil, cover and simmer for 30 minutes.

4. Next add the courgettes, trimmed and sliced, and pepper, de-seeded and sliced, to the pan. Stir, re-cover and cook for a further 20 minutes until the chicken is cooked through. Discard the lemon rind and bay leaves. Add sweetener and seasoning. Serve, sprinkled with olives and basil, with green vegetables and lemon wedges.

Cook's Notes
Part-boned chicken breasts are excellent for casseroles and stews as they combine the light tender meat of breast with the cooking capabilities of jointed cuts. If preferred, you can use skinned chicken quarters or bone-in skinned thighs.

Take care when preparing pumpkin, as the skin is often tough and it can be difficult to cut.

chicken kiev

The whole family will love this fabulous low-fat version of a family favourite. The low-fat fromage frais and Fry Light mean that the final dish is low in fat but not lessened in flavour.

Serves: 4

Preparation and cooking time: approximately 45 minutes

**4 x 142g/5oz boneless
skinless chicken breast
Salt and freshly ground
black pepper
2 garlic cloves
2 tbsp very low-fat natural
fromage frais
1 tbsp freshly chopped
parsley
2 level tbsp plus 2 level tsp
grated Parmesan cheese
1 small egg, beaten
28g/1oz golden
breadcrumbs
Fry Light
Lemon wedges to serve**

1. Preheat the oven to 190°C/375°F/Gas 5. Using a small sharp knife, slice lengthwise down the side of each chicken breast, taking care not to sever the flesh completely, to form a 'pocket'. Season the cavity.

2. Peel and crush the garlic cloves and mix with the fromage frais, the parsley and 2 tbsp Parmesan cheese. Spoon the mixture into each cavity and press together gently to seal. Secure the cavity by skewering with a cocktail stick and place the chicken breast on a sheet of baking parchment.

3. Brush the bottom side of each chicken breast with beaten egg and sprinkle lightly with half the breadcrumbs. Turn over and repeat with more egg and the remaining crumbs. Sprinkle the top lightly with the remaining Parmesan cheese.

4. Transfer to a baking sheet and spray with ten applications of Fry Light. Bake for 25-30 minutes until lightly golden and cooked through.

5. Serve with the lemon wedges accompanied by salad or green vegetables.

chicken korma

Curry has overtaken fish and chips as our favourite national dish, but high-fat sauces make take-out versions bad news for slimmers. However, this delicious low-fat recipe gives all the flavour with a fraction of the fat.

Serves: 4
Preparation time: approximately
15 minutes
Cooking time: approximately
30 minutes

227g/8oz onions
2.5cm/1in piece root ginger
3 cloves garlic
142ml/¼pt chicken stock,
made with Bovril
681g/1½lb boneless, skinless
chicken breasts
1 tbsp ground coriander
1 cinnamon stick, broken
5 cardamom pods,
lightly crushed
1 tsp salt
Ground black pepper
Juice of 1 small lemon
28g/1oz block creamed
coconut, grated
142g/5oz very low-fat
natural yogurt
14g/½oz toasted flaked
almonds
2 tbsp freshly chopped
coriander

1. Peel and roughly chop the onions, ginger and garlic. Place in a blender or food processor and blend for a few seconds to form a smooth paste. Transfer to a frying pan and add the stock. Bring to the boil and simmer gently for 5 minutes, stirring until tender.

2. Wash and pat dry the chicken breasts and cut into 4cm/1½in pieces. Add the chicken to the onion mixture and cook, stirring, for a further 5 minutes until the chicken is coloured all over. Stir in all the spices, seasoning and lemon juice. Add the coconut and cook gently, stirring occasionally, for 10 minutes.

3. Gradually add the yogurt, a spoonful at a time, stirring continuously, to blend into the mixture. Cook for a further minute until thick. Pour in 142ml/¼pt water. Bring to the boil and simmer gently for 15-20 minutes, stirring occasionally, until tender and cooked through.

4. Discard the cinnamon stick and cardamom pods. Transfer to a warm serving plate. Sprinkle with flaked almonds and chopped coriander and serve immediately with lemon wedges.

Cook's Notes
The sauce will thicken upon standing.

If you don't have a blender or food processor, simply chop the onion, ginger and garlic very finely, but the texture of the finished dish will be less smooth.

chicken with peaches
and raspberries

This chicken dish is a colourful and tasty combination of fruit and meat with a really summery feel. You can serve it hot, or cold as part of a salad.

Serves: 4

Preparation and cooking time: approximately 50 minutes

4 x 142g/5oz boneless skinless chicken fillets
Salt and freshly ground black pepper
2 tsp dried basil
Fry Light
4 large ripe peaches
Juice of 1 lemon
4 tbsp raspberry vinegar
1 level tbsp clear honey
113g/4oz raspberries, thawed if frozen
A few small basil leaves

1. Wash and pat dry the chicken breasts and season on both sides. Rub the dried basil on both sides of the chicken.

2. Lightly spray a non-stick griddle or large frying pan with Fry Light and heat until hot. Press the chicken into the pan using a fish slice. Cook for 2 minutes then turn over and cook for a further 2 minutes to seal the chicken. Lower the heat and cook the chicken for a further 20-25 minutes, turning frequently, or until tender and cooked through.

3. Meanwhile, wash and pat dry the peaches. Halve and stone and then halve again. Brush all over with lemon juice. Set aside.

4. Mix any remaining lemon juice with the vinegar and honey. Season and set aside.

5. Once the chicken is cooked, drain and keep warm. Reheat the griddle pan until hot and press the peach slices into the pan for a few seconds on each side to colour them lightly.

6. To serve, arrange the chicken with the peaches on warmed serving plates. Scatter a few raspberries on top and drizzle with the vinegar dressing. Sprinkle with a few basil leaves. Alternatively, allow the chicken and peaches to cool, chill and serve as a salad.

garlic chicken and vegetable pot roast

Once you've prepared this dish, you can put it in the oven and forget about it until it's ready to serve – it's a real meal in one.

Serves: 4
Preparation time: approximately
15 minutes
Cooking time: approximately
1 hour 30 minutes

2 small red peppers
2 small green peppers
227g/8oz shallots or
small onions
1 bulb fennel
1.4kg/3lb oven-ready chicken
Salt and freshly ground
black pepper
1 small lemon
142ml/¼pt chicken stock
made with Bovril
2 sprigs each of fresh thyme,
rosemary and tarragon
2 bay leaves
1 bulb garlic
1 tbsp fennel seeds

1. Preheat the oven to 180°C/350°F/Gas 4. Halve and de-seed the peppers and cut in half again. Place in the bottom of a large oval casserole with a tight-fitting lid. Peel and halve the shallots or onion and mix into the peppers. Trim the fennel and slice thickly. Place in the casserole.

2. Wash and pat dry the chicken and season inside and out. Halve the lemon and place inside the chicken. Place the chicken on top of the vegetables and pull some of the vegetables up around the sides of the chicken. Pour in the stock.

3. Tie the herbs together and place in the casserole. Break the bulb of garlic up and peel away the outer paper but do not peel the cloves. Scatter over the chicken and vegetables, and sprinkle with the fennel seeds.

4. Cover the casserole with a sheet of foil and then place the lid on top. Bake for 1¼-1½ hours until tender and cooked through and the juices run clear.

5. Drain the chicken and vegetables and place on a warmed serving platter. Remove the skin from the chicken before eating and serve with the garlic cloves and vegetables.

lemon chicken with artichokes

Artichokes have a unique flavour and somehow 'sweeten' everything you taste with them. They are rich in iron, mineral salts and vitamins.

Serves: 4

Preparation and cooking time: approximately 1 hour 15 minutes

4 x 227g/8oz part boned chicken breasts, skinned
Salt and freshly ground black pepper
1 tsp olive oil
2 medium red onions
1 medium lemon
1 large yellow pepper
142ml/¼pt dry white wine
426ml/¾pt chicken stock made with Bovril
113g/4oz button mushrooms
425g/15fl oz can artichoke hearts, drained
2 level tsp cornflour
1-2 tsp granulated artificial sweetener

1. Wash and pat dry the chicken breasts using kitchen paper and rub them with seasoning. Brush a ridged non-stick or plain frying pan with the oil and heat until hot. Press the chicken breasts into the pan for 1 minute on each side, over a high heat, to seal – if the pan is small, you may need to do two at a time. Drain them on kitchen paper and set aside.

2. Peel and quarter the onions and place in a large saucepan. Using a vegetable peeler, pare off four long strips of lemon rind into the pan. Squeeze the lemon juice and pour it over the onions, mixing well. Halve and de-seed the pepper, and then slice into thin strips and add it to the onions. Pour over the wine, bring to the boil, cover and simmer for 5 minutes.

3. Push the chicken breasts into the wine and vegetables and pour over the chicken stock. Bring the liquid back to the boil, cover the pan and simmer for 40 minutes.

4. Wipe and halve the mushrooms. Halve the artichoke hearts, stir both into the casserole and cook for a further 10 minutes until the chicken is tender and cooked through.

5. Remove the chicken from the saucepan with a slotted spoon and keep warm. Blend the cornflour with 2 tsp water and add to the stock and vegetables. Bring back to the boil, stirring until thickened.

6. Discard the lemon rind. Add sweetener and seasoning to taste. Serve the chicken with the lemon and vegetables spooned over.

thai green chicken curry

Here is another brilliant idea for a low-fat speedy supper with a hint of spice. From start to finish this tasty dish will only take you 30 minutes to prepare.

Serves: 4
Preparation and cooking time:
approximately 30 minutes

454g/1lb boneless, skinless chicken
2 cloves garlic
2 shallots
2.5cm/1in piece root ginger
1 green chilli
1 tsp coriander seeds
1 tsp salt
1 lime
2 x 15g/½oz packs fresh coriander
2 level tsp cornflour
28g/1oz block creamed coconut
113g/4oz fresh pineapple
1 small green pepper
1 small red chilli (optional)
Coriander sprig to garnish

1. Cut the chicken into 2.5cm/1in cubes and place in a bowl.

2. Peel the garlic, shallots and ginger. Halve and de-seed the chilli and lightly crush the coriander seeds. Place all these ingredients in a food processor or blender and add the salt.

3. Finely grate the lime rind, extract the juice and add to the garlic mixture along with one pack of fresh coriander. Process to form a smooth paste and then stir into the chicken along with the cornflour. Mix well.

4. Grate the coconut into a shallow pan and pour over 284ml/½pt water. Bring to the boil, stirring until dissolved. Add the chicken, mix well, bring back to the boil, cover and simmer for 15 minutes or until the chicken is cooked through.

5. Meanwhile, finely chop the pineapple and place in a small bowl. Halve, de-seed and finely chop the pepper and chilli, if using, and finely chop the remaining fresh coriander. Mix the pepper, chilli and coriander into the pineapple and chill until required.

6. Serve the chicken garnished with a sprig of fresh coriander, accompanied with the pineapple relish and green vegetables.

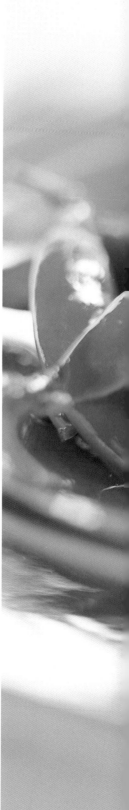

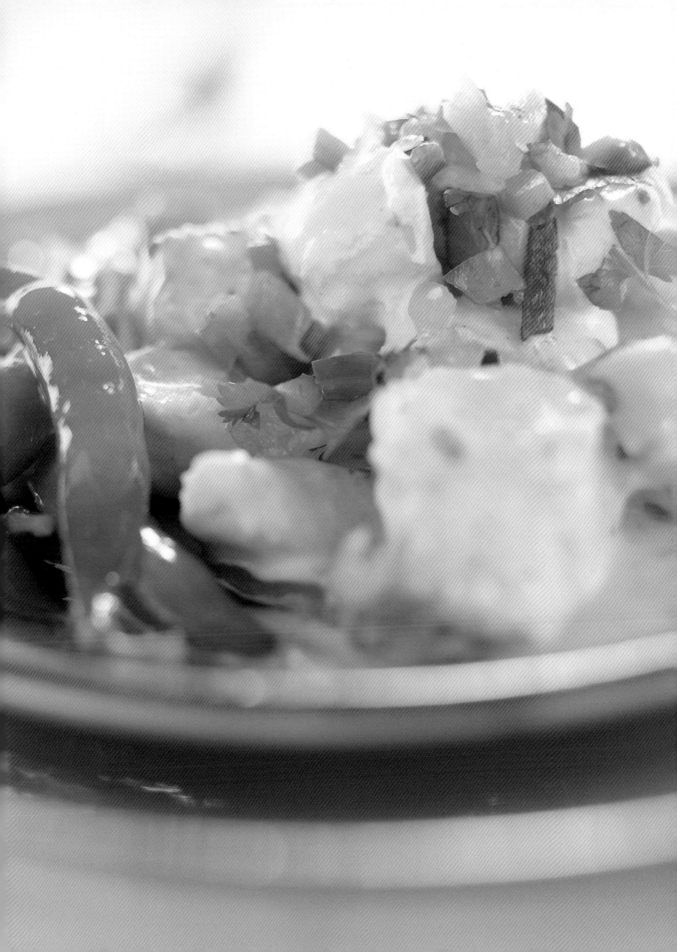

hot chicken sandwich

A sandwich with a twist – this dish is equally delicious barbecued or cooked in a griddle pan. To make the sandwich in this way, follow steps 1 to 4 below and cook in a hot non-stick griddle pan for 18-20 minutes, turning occasionally.

Serves: 4
Preparation and cooking time:
approximately 35 minutes

4 x 142g/5oz skinless,
boneless chicken breasts
1 medium courgette
2 medium tomatoes
2 garlic cloves
Salt and freshly ground
black pepper
Fry Light

1. Using a sharp knife, carefully slice each chicken breast widthwise through the middle, so that you end up with two flat pieces. Set aside.

2. Trim the courgette and slice thinly on the diagonal. Slice the tomatoes thinly. Peel the garlic cloves and slice them thinly as well.

3. Lay four pieces of chicken on a board and top with a layer of courgette, tomato and sliced garlic. Season well. Then place the other pieces of chicken on top. Tie with string or secure the 'sandwiches' together using skewers or cocktail sticks.

4. Spray each side lightly with Fry Light, place on hot coals and cook for 12-15 minutes, turning occasionally until golden and cooked. Serve hot.

mango duck with mustard mash

Tender lean bacon is wrapped around duck breasts before grilling to help prevent drying out during cooking. Keep the heat at a medium setting so that the duck cooks gradually and maintains its juiciness.

Serves: 4
Preparation time: approximately
15 minutes
Cooking time: approximately
1 hour

4 x 170g/6oz boneless duck breasts
Salt and freshly ground black pepper
2 level tbsp smooth mango chutney
6 rashers lean rindless unsmoked back bacon
340g/12oz carrots
340g/12oz swede
1 tsp mustard seeds, crushed
2 tbsp very low-fat natural fromage frais
2 spring onions, trimmed and chopped, to garnish

1. Remove the skin and any excess fat from the duck breasts. Season on both sides and spread the mango chutney all over.

2. Trim away any excess fat from the bacon and cut each rasher in half lengthwise. Wrap three strips around each duck breast.

3. Preheat the grill to a medium setting. Arrange the duck breasts on the grill rack and cook for 40 minutes, turning occasionally, or until tender, golden and cooked through.

4. Meanwhile, peel and finely chop the carrots and swede. Place in a saucepan and cover with water. Add a pinch of salt and bring to the boil. Cook for 8-10 minutes until tender and cooked through. Drain well and mash using a potato masher or fork.

5. Stir the mustard seeds and fromage frais into the mashed vegetables and adjust the seasoning. Keep warm until required.

6. To serve, drain the duck and serve with the mash, sprinkled with chopped spring onion to garnish.

kleftico-style lamb steaks

Usually this Greek dish is made using a joint of lamb which is slowly cooked in a clay oven. But it works just as well using lamb steaks, and with this method they come out of the oven beautifully tender and moist.

Serves: 4
Preparation time: approximately 10 minutes
Cooking time: approximately 1 hour 30 minutes

2 medium red onions
2 garlic cloves
2 tbsp lemon juice
4 medium tomatoes
A few sprigs fresh rosemary
4 x 142g/5oz lean lamb steaks
Salt and freshly ground black pepper
Fresh rosemary to garnish

1. Preheat the oven to 180°C/350°F/Gas 4. Peel the onions and garlic. Slice the onions into thin wedges and toss in the lemon juice. Thinly slice the garlic. Remove the stalks from the tomatoes and cut into quarters.

2. Arrange the onions, garlic and tomatoes in the base of a sealable casserole dish and sprinkle with rosemary sprigs.

3. Trim away any excess fat from the lamb steaks and season on both sides. Arrange on top of the vegetables. Cover with a layer of foil and then the lid. Bake in the oven for about 1½ hours or until very tender.

4. Drain and serve garnished with fresh rosemary, and accompanied with green vegetables or a crisp Greek-style salad.

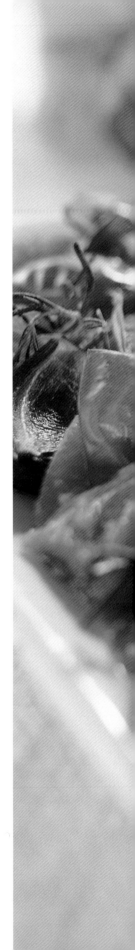

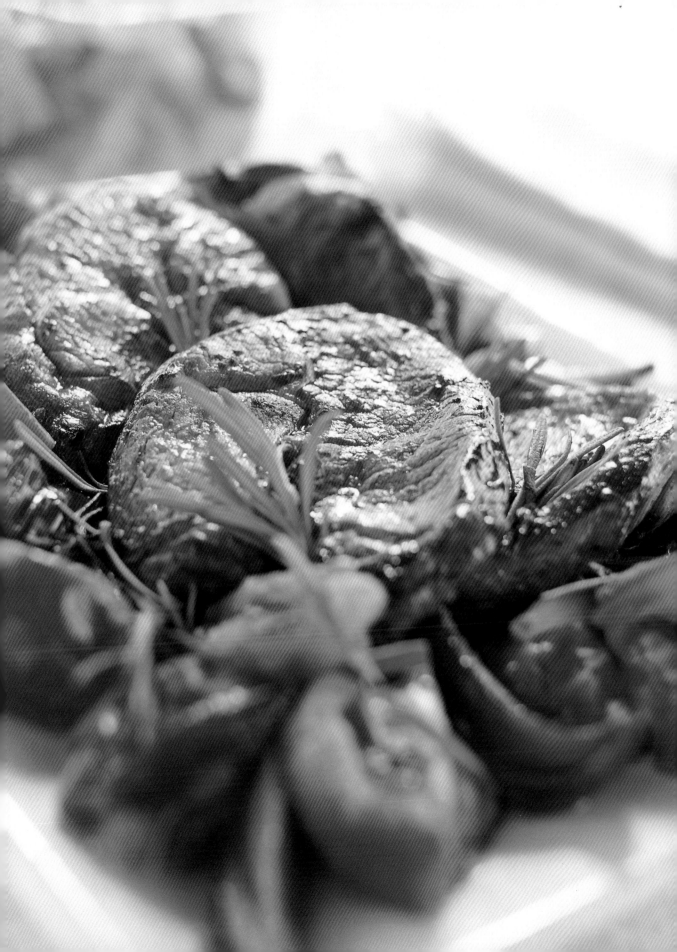

roast lamb with a curried crust

This dish cooks in its own juices so you don't need any fat. The lid needs to be secure and well fitting in order to prevent any steam escaping.

Serves: 4
Preparation time: approximately
15 minutes plus marinating and
standing
Cooking time: approximately
2 hours

1.3kg/2¾lb half leg of lamb
2.5cm/1in piece root ginger
4 garlic cloves
1 medium onion
1 fresh green chilli
170g/6oz low-fat natural
yogurt
2 tbsp mild curry powder
1 tsp salt
1 ripe large mango
15g/½oz packet fresh
coriander
lemon wedges to garnish

1. Preheat the oven to 180°C/350°F/Gas 4. Remove all visible fat from the lamb and lay on a board. Using a small sharp knife, make deep incisions all over the lamb – make them as deep as possible, trying to slice to the bone. Place the lamb in a deep casserole with a lid.

2. Peel and roughly chop the ginger, garlic and onion and place in a food processor or blender. Halve and de-seed the chilli. Roughly chop and add to the food processor along with the yogurt, curry powder and salt. Blend for a few seconds until smooth.

3. Spoon the spiced yogurt over the lamb and spread well to completely coat the surface of the meat. Cover and chill for 2 hours.

4. Remove the covering, and cover the dish with foil. Fit the lid and bake in the oven for 1¾-2 hours or until very tender and cooked through. Stand for 10 minutes.

5. While the lamb is standing, peel the mango and slice down either side of the smooth, flat, central stone. Slice or chop the flesh. Cover and chill until required. Roughly chop the coriander, cover and chill until required.

6. To serve, drain the lamb and place on a warmed serving platter. Scatter with chopped coriander and serve with the mango and wedges of lemon.

caribbean pork

Pork is a rich meat and is therefore complemented by being served with fruit. Baby pineapples are particularly tender and sweet, but larger ripe varieties work just as well. A pineapple should smell sweet through its skin when ripe.

Serves: 4
Preparation time: approximately
15 minutes plus chilling
Cooking time: approximately
15 minutes

4 x 142g/5oz lean boneless
pork steaks or chops
Salt and freshly ground
black pepper
1 level tbsp dark brown
sugar
1 tbsp dark rum
3 tbsp unsweetened
pineapple juice
1 baby (queen) pineapple or
½ medium pineapple
1 large red pepper
Fry Light

1. Trim away any excess fat from the pork and season on both sides. Place in a shallow dish. Mix the brown sugar with the rum and pineapple juice and pour over the pork. Cover and chill for 30 minutes.

2. Meanwhile, peel the pineapple and cut into 1cm/½in thick slices; core if necessary. Halve and de-seed the pepper, cut into thick, flat wedges. Set aside.

3. Spray a non-stick griddle or large frying pan with Fry Light and heat until hot. Drain the pork, reserving the juices, and press into the pan using a fish slice and cook for 1 minute to seal. Turn over and cook on a high heat for a further 1 minute. Lower the heat and continue to cook for a further 7-8 minutes, turning frequently, until golden, tender and cooked through. Drain.

4. Toss the pineapple and peppers in the reserved juices and cook the peppers in the pan for 2-3 minutes until tender, and the pineapple for about 30 seconds on each side. Drain.

5. Serve the pork steaks with some pineapple and pepper. Accompany with freshly cooked vegetables.

redcurrant lamb with leek and swede mash

A really tasty but quick way to serve lamb steaks. Lamb chops are just as good in this recipe; simply make sure you trim off any visible fat.

Serves: 4
Preparation and cooking time:
approximately 30 minutes

4 level tbsp redcurrant jelly
1 tsp dried rosemary
Garlic salt and freshly
ground black pepper
4 x 100g/3½oz (approximate
weight) lean boneless lamb
leg steaks
454g/1lb swede
454g/1lb leeks
142ml/¼pt vegetable stock
1 tbsp very low-fat natural
fromage frais

1. Melt 2 tbsp of the redcurrant jelly in a small saucepan and add the rosemary and seasoning.

2. Preheat the grill to a medium/hot setting. Trim lamb if necessary and arrange of a grill rack. Brush on the redcurrant mixture over the lamb and grill for 7 minutes. Turn, brush again and cook for a further 7-8 minutes or until cooked to your liking.

3. Meanwhile, peel the swede and cut into small cubes. Place in a saucepan and cover with water. Bring to the boil and cook for 8-10 minutes until softened. Drain well.

4. Trim the leeks and rinse under running water. Slice and place in a saucepan with the stock. Bring to the boil, cover and simmer for 5 minutes until tender. Drain, reserving the cooking liquid.

5. Place the swede and leeks in a bowl and mash with a potato masher. Season and mix in the fromage frais. Set aside and keep warm.

6. In a saucepan, melt the remaining redcurrant jelly and blend in the reserved leek cooking liquid. Bring to the boil and boil rapidly for 2 minutes to reduce slightly.

7. To serve, pile some swede and leek mash on a warmed serving plate, top with a lamb steak and spoon over a little redcurrant jelly sauce. Serve with a selection of steamed vegetables.

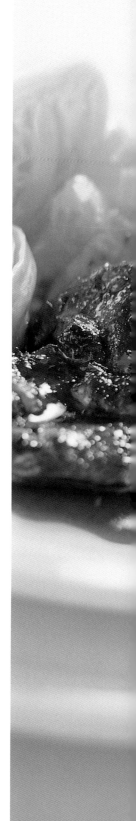

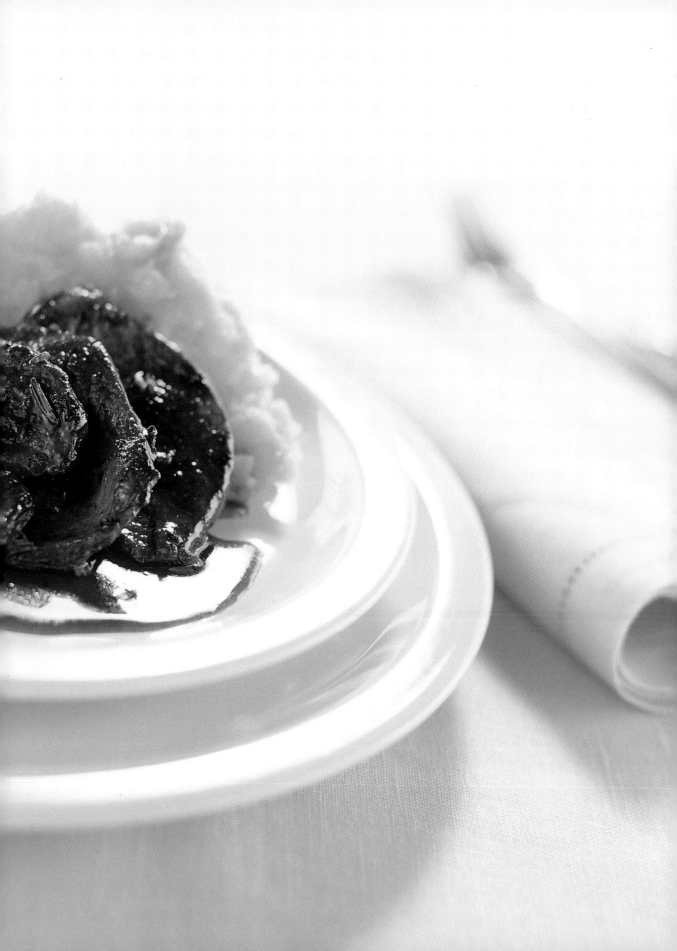

mustard pork steaks with red cabbage

This dish is perfect for winter days accompanied by broccoli, carrot and mashed swede. But it is equally delicious served with a generous salad.

Serves: 4
Preparation and cooking time:
approximately 30 minutes

½ medium red cabbage
2 red onions
28g/1oz low-fat spread
142ml/¼pt red wine vinegar
1 tsp ground cinnamon
Salt and freshly ground
black pepper
1-2 tbsp granular artificial
sweetener
4 x 113g/4oz lean boneless
pork steaks
2 level tbsp wholegrain
mustard

1. Trim the cabbage and finely shred. Peel and finely chop the onions.

2. In a large saucepan, melt the low-fat spread over a low heat. Stir in the cabbage and onion and mix well to coat. Add the vinegar, cinnamon, seasoning and 4 tbsp water. Bring to the boil, cover and simmer for 15 minutes. Stir in the artificial sweetener to taste.

3. Meanwhile, trim the pork if necessary. Season to taste and spread on both sides with mustard.

4. Preheat the grill to a medium/hot setting. Arrange the pork steaks on a grill rack and cook for 7 minutes. Turn over and grill for a further 7-8 minutes or until cooked through.

5. To serve, drain the cabbage and pile on to a warmed serving plate. Top with a pork steak and serve. Accompany it with broccoli, carrots and mashed swede – perfect comfort food for winter days!

turkey satay with peanut sauce

Turkey is a very lean meat so it is ideal to serve with a rich sauce like this one. Satay is also made with chicken, beef and pork. The peanut sauce tastes good with grilled or baked vegetables.

Serves: 4
Preparation time: approximately
20 minutes plus marinating
Cooking time: approximately
12 minutes

**454g/1lb lean boneless
skinless turkey
1 shallot or small onion
1 garlic clove
2.5cm/1in piece root ginger
Juice of 1 lime or ½ small
lemon
1 tbsp five spice powder
2 tbsp dark soy sauce
14g/½oz block creamed
coconut
2 level tbsp crunchy peanut
butter
2 level tsp clear honey
¼ tsp garlic salt
½ tsp hot chilli powder
½ tsp ground cumin**

1. Slice the turkey into thin shreds about 6mm/¼in thick. Place in a shallow bowl. Peel the shallot and garlic and finely chop. Peel and grate the ginger. Mix into the turkey along with the lime juice, five spice powder and soy sauce. Mix well, cover and chill for 2 hours to allow the flavours to develop.

2. Soak eight bamboo skewers in cold water for 30 minutes. Grate the coconut into a small saucepan and pour in 142ml/¼pt water. Blend in the peanut butter and honey. Bring to the boil and simmer for 5 minutes until thickened. Remove from the heat and stir in the remaining ingredients and the remaining soy sauce. Set aside.

3. Drain the skewers and thread the turkey on to them in 'S' shapes to within 2.5cm/1in of the ends.

4. Preheat the grill to a hot setting. Arrange the skewers on the grill rack and cook for 5-6 minutes, brushing with any remaining marinade, until tender and cooked through.

5. To serve, heat up the sauce and transfer to a small serving dish. Drain the satay and serve with lime or lemon wedges and a crisp salad.

pork and herb meatballs with ratatouille sauce

Tender morsels of herby lean pork are grilled and served on a bed of rich and colourful Mediterranean vegetables. Use minced beef, lamb or chicken as an alternative if preferred.

Serves: 4
Preparation time: approximately
20 minutes plus chilling
Cooking time: approximately
20 minutes

4 spring onions
454g/1lb extra lean minced
pork
1 tsp dried mixed herbs
Salt and freshly ground
black pepper
1 small onion
1 small yellow pepper
1 small courgette
1 baby aubergine
1 bay leaf
397g/14oz can chopped
tomatoes with garlic
2 tbsp freshly chopped
parsley

1. Trim and finely chop the white and green parts of the spring onions. Place in a mixing bowl and add the minced pork, dried herbs and plenty of seasoning. Mix well to combine and then divide into twenty portions. Form into small balls and place on a plate lined with baking parchment. Cover and chill for 30 minutes.

2. Meanwhile prepare the sauce. Peel the onion and chop finely. Halve and de-seed the pepper and chop finely. Trim the courgette and aubergine and chop finely. Place in a saucepan along with the bay leaf and chopped tomatoes. Season well, bring to the boil and simmer for 10 minutes until tender. Set aside until ready to serve.

3. Preheat the grill to a medium/hot setting. Arrange the meatballs on the grill rack and cook for 8-10 minutes, turning frequently or until golden and cooked through. Drain well.

4. Reheat the sauce until piping hot, discard the bay leaf and serve the meatballs with the sauce, sprinkled with chopped parsley.

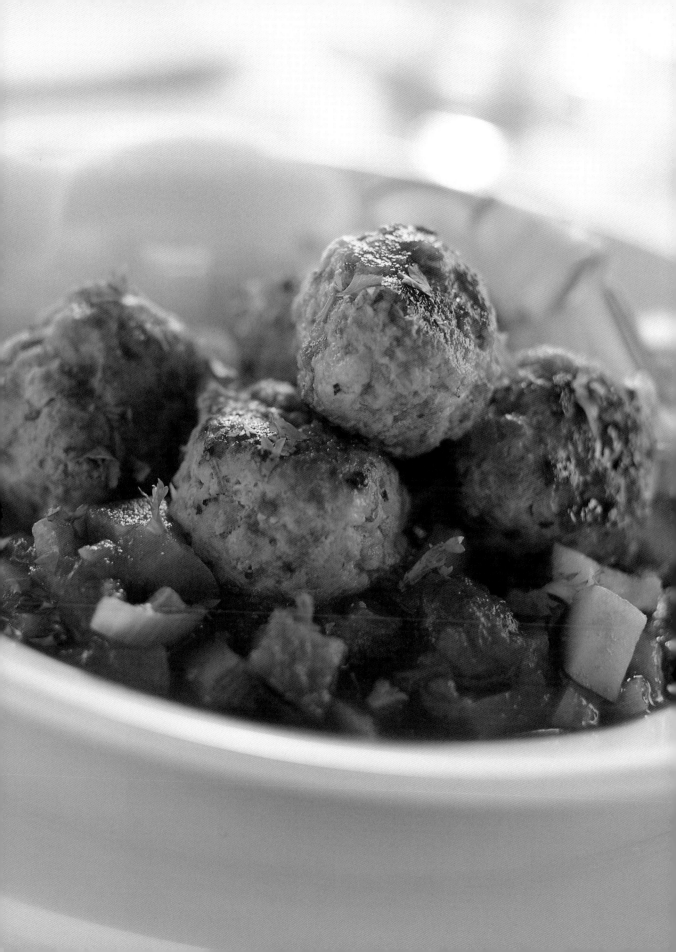

corned beef hash

Corned beef hash has always been a firm favourite — it's a great store cupboard standby. Serve with a jacket potato and mixed salad for a speedy lunch.

Serves: 4
Preparation and cooking time:
approximately 20 minutes.

1 medium onion
1 small green pepper
142ml/½pt beef stock made
with Bovril
340g/12oz can corned beef
397g/14oz can chopped
tomatoes with garlic
200g/7oz pack cooked
beetroot in natural juice
salt and freshly ground black
pepper
4 tbsp very low-fat natural
fromage frais
2 tbsp freshly chopped
chives

1. Peel and finely slice the onion. Halve, de-seed and chop the pepper. Place in a saucepan along with the beef stock. Bring to the boil, cover and simmer for approximately 5 minutes.

2. Meanwhile, remove any excess fat from the corned beef and cut into bite sized chunks. Carefully stir into the onion and peppers, along with the chopped tomatoes, taking care not to break up the corned beef, and heat through for 3-4 minutes.

3. Drain the beetroot and cut into small pieces. Gently stir into the corned beef mixture along with plenty of seasoning. Heat through, stirring gently, for a further 1-2 minutes until piping hot.

4. Serve each portion with a spoonful of fromage frais on top, sprinkled with fresh chopped chives and more black pepper if liked.

steak and mushroom pie

Don't be put off by the long cooking time on this recipe – the preparation time is quick. We guarantee that the rich flavour and crisp pastry make it well worth the wait!

Serves: 4
Preparation time: approximately
15 minutes plus cooling
Cooking time: approximately
2 hours 10 minutes

1 medium onion
681g/1½lb lean cubed
braising steak
1 level tbsp cornflour
2 bay leaves
Salt and freshly ground
black pepper
284ml/½pt beef stock
227g/8oz closed cup
mushrooms
3 x 28g/1oz sheets filo
pastry
1 medium egg, beaten

1. Peel and slice the onion and place in a pan. Remove all visible fat from the steak, toss in the cornflour and add it to the pan with the bay leaves and seasoning. Add the stock and about 142ml/¼pt water to just cover the beef. Bring to the boil, cover and simmer for 1½ hours until the beef is tender. Cool, then discard the bay leaves.

2. Preheat the oven to 220°C/425°F/Gas 7. Quarter the mushrooms and place in a 908ml/2pt pie dish. Add the beef and onions using a slotted spoon, and pour over about 200ml/7floz of the cooking liquid to come halfway up the dish. The meat will come to the top, but once the mushrooms cook down the level will sink.

3. Brush each sheet of pastry with egg, lightly scrunch up and place on top of the meat, pulling the sheets out to make sure all the meat is covered. Brush generously with egg and bake for 20 minutes. Lower the heat to 180°C/350°F/Gas 4 and continue to cook for a further 20 minutes until golden and hot. Serve with green vegetables.

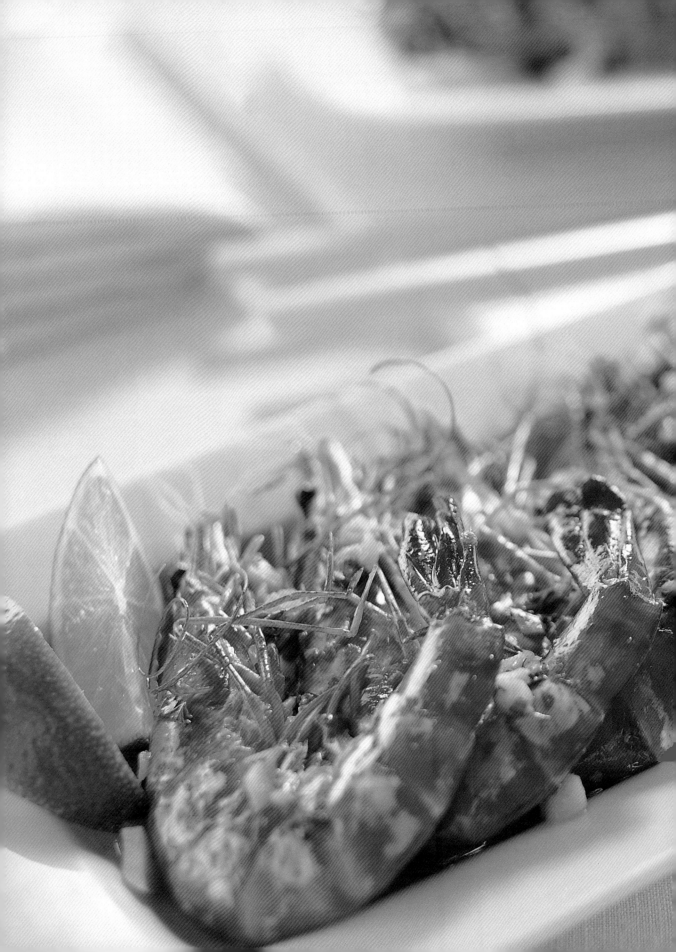

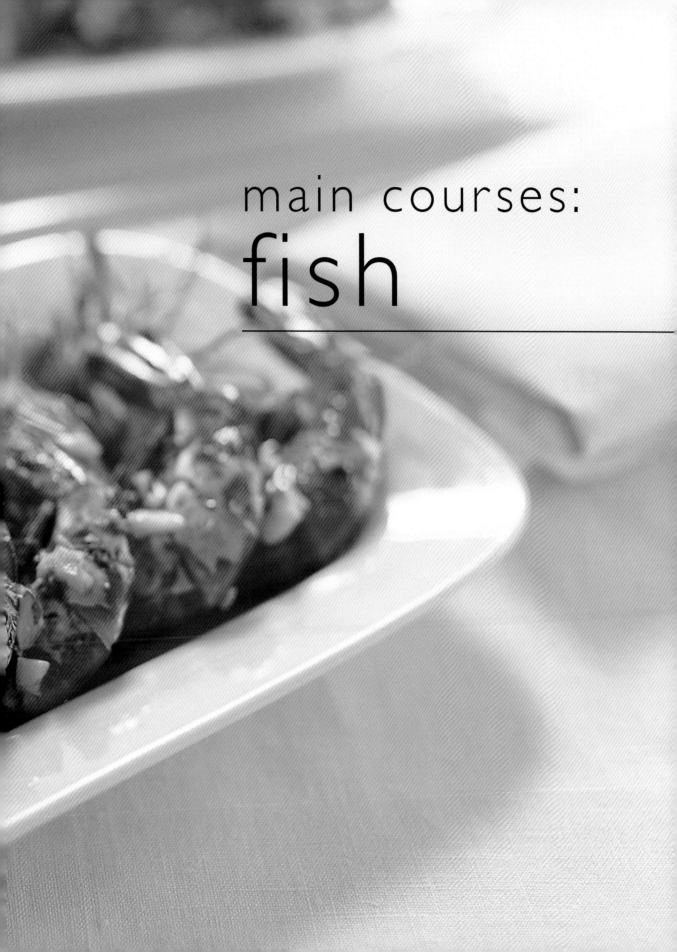

main courses:
fish

cajun griddled fish

Way down south in New Orleans and Louisiana, both fish and chicken are 'blackened' in a butter and spice crust. This lighter version is very tasty, and is so easy to prepare and cook – try it on the barbecue in the summer.

Serves: 4
Preparation time: approximately
10 minutes
Cooking time: approximately
5 minutes

1 tbsp paprika
½ tsp dried onion powder
½ tsp garlic salt
½ tsp ground cumin
½ tsp cayenne pepper
½ tsp ground black pepper
1 tsp dried thyme
4 x 170g/6oz skinless white
fish fillets about 1cm/½in
thick, such as cod, halibut or
sea bass
Juice of 1 lime or ½ small
lemon
Fry Light
Lime wedges and fresh
thyme to garnish

1. In a small bowl, mix together the paprika, onion powder, garlic salt, cumin, cayenne, pepper and thyme.

2. Wash and pat dry the fish fillets and sprinkle with lime or lemon juice. Spread a thin layer of the spice mixture over both sides of the fish, making sure they are completely coated.

3. Spray a non-stick griddle or large frying pan with Fry Light and heat until very hot and press the fish fillets into the pan using a fish slice – there will be a hiss and some smoke. Cook for 2 minutes until richly golden and slightly blackened, then turn over and cook for a further 2 minutes until tender and cooked through.

4. Drain and serve with lime wedges and fresh thyme sprigs sprinkled over. Accompany with a crisp salad.

cod in parsley sauce

An old family favourite has been given a makeover here, reducing the fat levels. But this cod in parsley sauce will still tantalise your tastebuds.

Serves: 4

Preparation and cooking time: approximately 20 minutes

4 x 170g/6oz skinless thick cod fillets or cod loin
I tsp finely grated lemon rind
Juice of I small lemon
Freshly ground black pepper
8 bay leaves
2 level tsp cornflour
142ml/¼pt skimmed milk
142ml/¼pt fish or vegetable stock
113g/4oz very low-fat natural fromage frais
4 tbsp freshly chopped parsley

1. Bring a large saucepan of water to the boil. Place the fish in a steaming compartment, colander or large sieve. Sprinkle with lemon rind, juice and black pepper. Add the bay leaves, cover and steam for 7-8 minutes until cooked through.

2. Meanwhile blend the cornflour with a little of the milk to form a paste. Pour into a saucepan with the rest of the milk and the stock. Bring to the boil, stirring, and cook gently for 1 minute until thickened.

3. Remove from the heat and cool for 5 minutes. Stir in the fromage frais and parsley. Season to taste and return to the heat. Heat through over a low heat until hot – do not allow to boil.

4. Drain the fish and discard the bay leaves. Place on warmed plates and spoon over the sauce. Accompany with fresh vegetables.

pan-cooked prawns with garlic and vermouth

Quite an unusual way to cook prawns, this dish makes a delicious starter or main course. As it only takes 10 minutes to prepare it's an ideal dish to serve when entertaining or if you are in a hurry.

Serves: 4
Preparation and cooking time:
approximately 10 minutes

4 garlic cloves
24 unshelled large raw prawns
2 tsp olive oil
Juice of 1 lemon
2 tbsp dry white vermouth
Salt and freshly ground black pepper
2 tbsp freshly chopped parsley

1. Peel and slice the garlic. Wash the prawns and pat dry with absorbent kitchen paper.

2. Heat the oil in a wok or large frying pan until hot and add the garlic then the prawns in a single layer – cook the prawns in two batches if necessary, turning frequently. Stir-fry for 2 minutes until coated with the oil. Add the lemon juice and simmer, stirring, for a further 2 minutes until all the prawns are pink.

3. Sprinkle with vermouth and season to taste. Sprinkle with parsley and serve immediately.

Cook's Notes
Large prawns like these are expensive but they have a delicious taste and make a stunning course for a special dinner.

You can use raw unpeeled tiger prawns as a less expensive alternative, and you will need to allow about 8-10 per person.

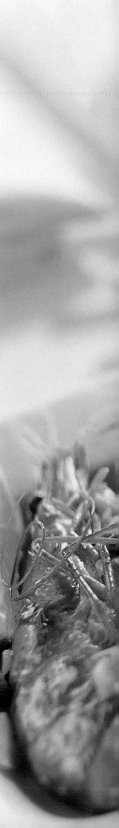

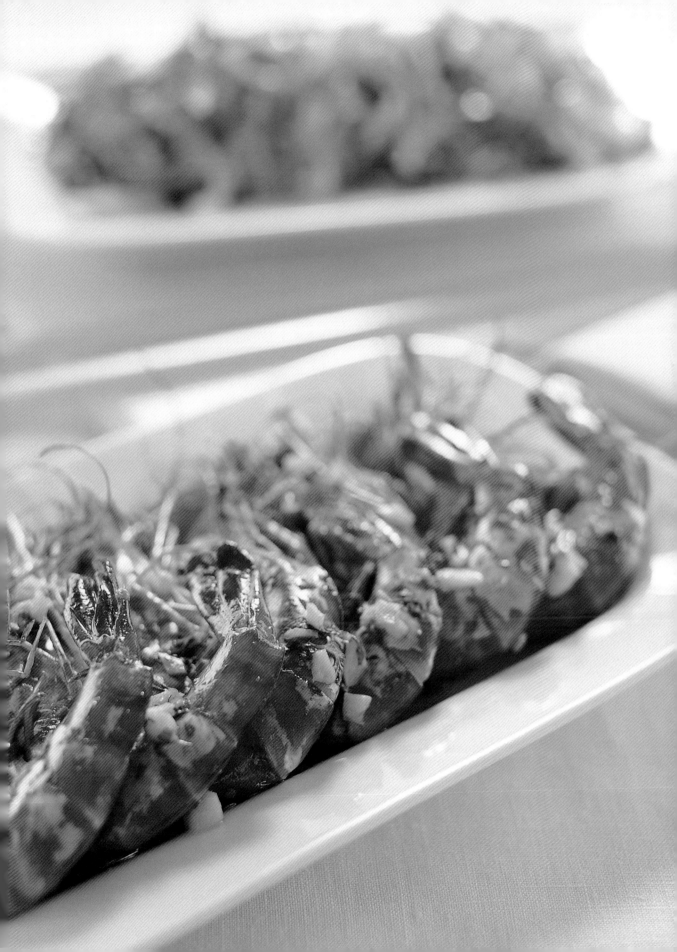

greek fish wrapped in vine leaves

Try this delicious recipe when barbecuing, or it's equally tasty grilled. To help you on your way, look out for preserved vine leaves in brine in vacuum packs in your local supermarket or delicatessen.

Serves: 4
Preparation and cooking time:
approximately 30 minutes
plus chilling

4 x 170g/6oz firm white fish
fillets such as monkfish, cod,
halibut
1 garlic clove, peeled and
crushed
1 small red onion, peeled
and finely chopped
4 tbsp lemon juice
½ tsp finely grated lemon
rind
28g/1oz pitted black olives
in brine, drained and sliced
1 tbsp freshly chopped
oregano or 1 tsp dried
Salt and freshly ground
black pepper
Approximately 16 large
preserved vine leaves,
drained and rinsed

1. Place the fish in a shallow dish and sprinkle with the garlic, onion, lemon juice and rind, olives, oregano and seasoning. Cover and chill for 30 minutes.

2. Drain fish and place each piece on two overlapping vine leaves. Wrap up, using two more leaves to cover it completely (you may need more). Secure with string if necessary to hold the leaves in place.

3. Place the fish steaks in a wire barbecue basket. Place over medium/hot coals and cook for 15-20 minutes, turning once until the fish is cooked through. Do not let the fish overcook. Alternatively, place on a grill rack under a medium/hot grill and cook as above.

Cook's Note

If preferred, you can use cabbage leaves. Simply blanch them in boiling water for 4-5 minutes until just tender. Drain and cool in cold water.

monkfish and bacon kebabs

Monkfish is a very firm white fish ideal for chunky kebabs. Here it is wrapped in bacon for flavour and to help it retain moisture during cooking.

Serves: 4
Preparation time: approximately
20 minutes
Cooking time: approximately
10 minutes

1 medium red onion
1 tbsp lemon juice
1 small red pepper
1 small orange or yellow
pepper
454g/1lb monkfish fillets
Freshly ground black pepper
4 tbsp freshly chopped
parsley
4 lean rindless rashers back
bacon

1. Peel the onion and cut into thin wedges. Separate the layers and toss in the lemon juice. Halve and de-seed the peppers and cut into 2.5cm/1in pieces.

2. Wash and pat dry the monkfish and cut into 2cm/¾in chunks. Place in a bowl and season with black pepper. Toss in 3 tbsp chopped parsley and mix well so that the fish is coated.

3. Removed all visible fat from the bacon and cut each bacon rasher lengthwise into sufficient thin strips to pieces of fish. Wrap a strip around each piece of fish and thread on to eight skewers alternating with pieces of onion and peppers.

4. Preheat the grill to a medium/hot setting. Arrange the skewers on the grill rack and cook for 4-5 minutes on each side until tender and cooked through. Drain and serve sprinkled with remaining parsley.

Cook's Note
If you want to use bamboo skewers, soak them for 30 minutes in cold water before you use them. This will prevent the skewers burning too much. Alternatively, cover up the ends with small pieces of foil.

plaice and salmon rolls

Rolls of tender plaice fillets with luscious smoked salmon surrounded by a delicate green watercress sauce, make an elegant dish, ideal for entertaining.

Serves: 4
Preparation time: approximately
20 minutes
Cooking time: approximately
20 minutes

4 x 113g/4oz skinless plaice fillets
113g/4oz smoked salmon
57g/2oz low-fat soft cheese with garlic and herbs
1 tbsp freshly chopped dill
4 tbsp lemon juice
Salt and freshly ground black pepper
170g/6oz very low-fat natural fromage frais
28g/1oz watercress
2 tbsp freshly chopped parsley
1 tsp finely grated lemon rind
Watercress and chopped dill to garnish

1. Preheat the oven to 190°C/375°F/Gas 5. Halve the salmon fillets lengthwise and lay strips of smoked salmon over the skinned side of each fillet, trimming as necessary.

2. Soften the cheese by lightly beating it and then spread a little over the smoked salmon. Sprinkle with some dill and carefully roll up from the narrow, tail, end.

3. Place them side by side, seam side down, in a shallow baking dish and sprinkle with 2 tbsp lemon juice. Season and cover with foil. Bake in the oven for 15-20 minutes, until tender and just cooked through.

4. Meanwhile, place the fromage frais, watercress, remaining lemon juice, parsley and half the lemon rind in a food processor or blender and blend until smooth. Cover and chill until required.

5. To serve, drain the fish and place on warmed serving plates and sprinkle with remaining lemon rind. Season with black pepper and garnish with watercress and chopped dill.

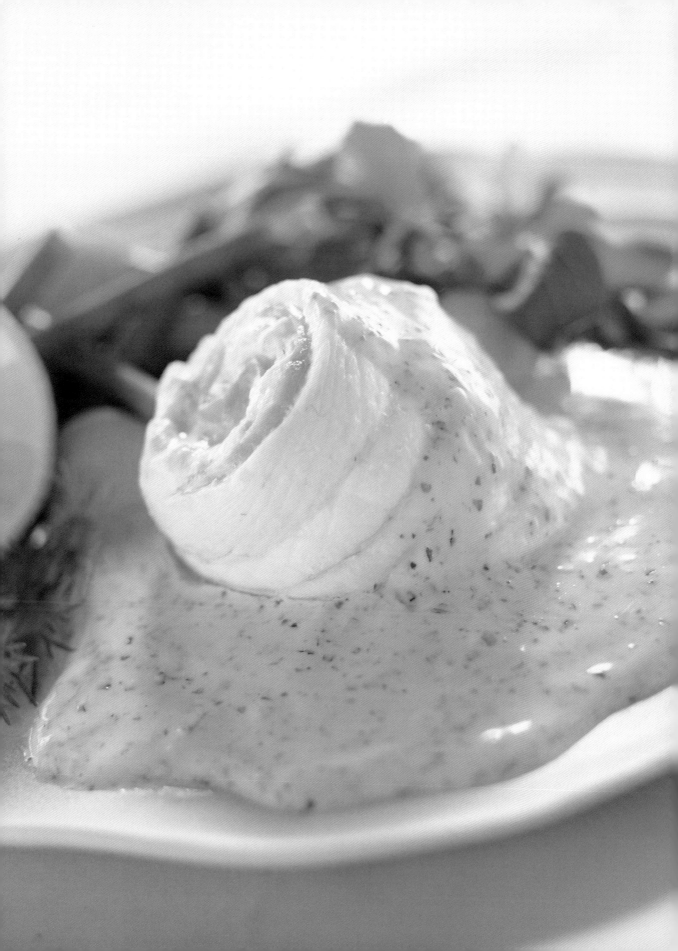

ribbon trout

This colourful dish looks really pretty and smells superb. For the best flavour, use rainbow or brown trout; both are equally delicious.

Serves: 4
Preparation and cooking time:
approximately 50 minutes

4 x 227g/8oz whole trout,
cleaned
Salt and freshly ground
black pepper
2 medium carrots
2 medium courgettes
1 small leek
2.5cm/1in piece root ginger
2 tbsp lemon juice

1. Preheat the oven to 190°C/375°F/Gas 5. Wash the trout inside and out and pat dry using absorbent kitchen paper. Season the insides of the fish and set aside.

2. Trim and peel the carrots and trim the courgettes. Using a vegetable peeler or cheese slicer, slice off 12 'ribbons' from one carrot and one courgette. Bring a saucepan of water to the boil and blanch the ribbons in the water for 30 seconds to soften. Drain and rinse in cold water. Set to one side.

3. Finely shred or grate the remaining carrot and courgette and place in a bowl. Trim and wash the leek and then finely shred. Peel and grate the ginger. Mix into the other vegetables along with 1 tbsp lemon juice.

4. Pack a sufficient amount of vegetables into each fish cavity. Wrap three ribbons of carrot and three of courgette, overlapping, around each trout and place on a baking sheet lined with baking parchment. Spoon over remaining lemon juice and bake for 25-30 minutes, until cooked through. Serve immediately with green vegetables.

Cook's Note
This attractive way of cooking fish will also work well with fish steaks. Simply slice the flesh in half through the middle, place the vegetables on one half and sandwich back together. Then wrap the fish in the vegetable ribbons and bake as above.

salmon florentine

An elegant version of the classic poached egg dish. Salmon and spinach is a winning combination, and this is a quick and suitably light dish for supper-time.

Serves: 4
Preparation time: approximately
15 minutes
Cooking time: approximately
15 minutes

4 x 142g/5oz fillets skinless salmon
2 bay leaves
142ml/¼pt dry white wine
Salt and freshly ground black pepper
454g/1lb baby spinach leaves
2 large leeks
113g/4oz very low-fat natural fromage frais
½ tsp ground nutmeg

1. Wash and pat dry the salmon and place in a shallow frying pan with a lid. Add the bay leaves and pour over the wine and 142ml/¼pt of cold water. Season and bring to the boil. Cover and simmer gently for 7-8 minutes until just cooked through. Turn off the heat and allow to stand until required.

2. Meanwhile, rinse the spinach and pack into a large saucepan while still wet. Trim the leeks and split lengthwise. Rinse under cold running water to flush out any trapped earth. Shake well to remove excess water and then shred finely. Reserving a little shredded leek for garnish, mix the remaining into the wet spinach.

3. Cover and place on a medium heat for 4-5 minutes until wilted – the vegetables will cook in the steam. Don't have the heat too high otherwise the spinach may stick on the bottom of the pan. Drain well by pressing against the side of the colander or sieve to remove as much water as possible.

4. Transfer the spinach to a blender or food processor and add the fromage frais and plenty of seasoning. Blend for a few seconds until smooth.

5. To serve, divide the spinach between warmed serving plates. Drain the salmon and place a piece on top of each portion of spinach. Dust with ground nutmeg and sprinkle with reserved leek to garnish.

Cook's Note
Replace the wine with fish or vegetable stock if you prefer.

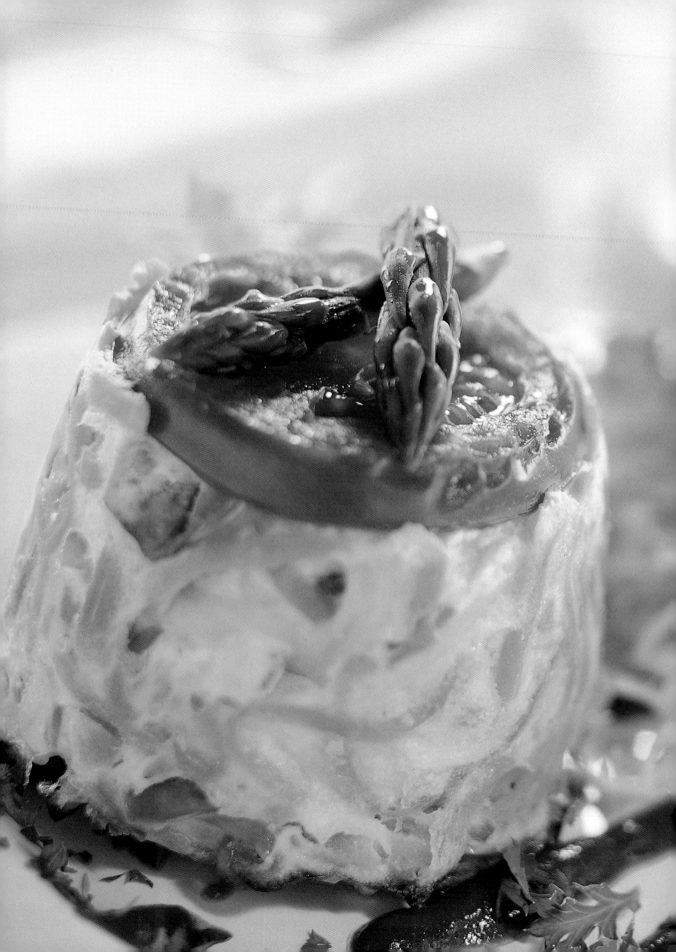

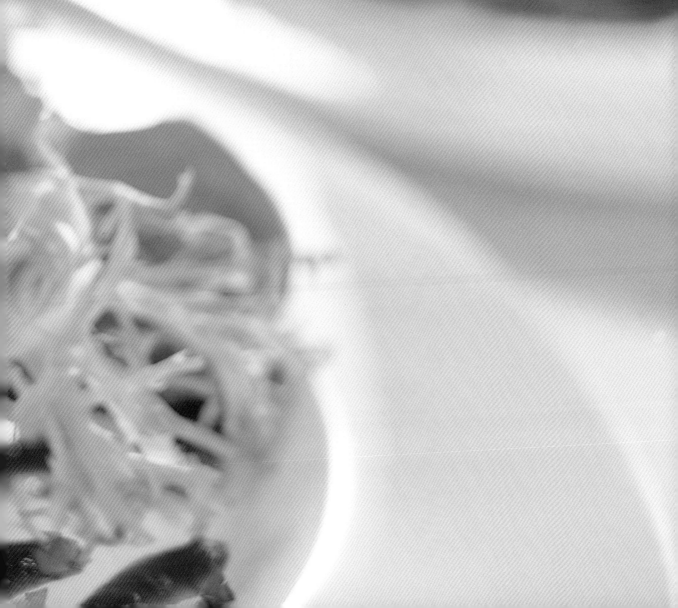

main courses:
vegetarian

macaroni cheese stuffed peppers

You can use any coloured peppers for this dish, but the red and yellow varieties are particularly sweet. The chilli powder adds a touch of spice, but for a milder flavour replace with ground paprika.

Serves: 4
Preparation time: approximately
15 minutes
Cooking time: approximately
35 minutes

4 large red peppers
Salt and freshly ground
black pepper
17g/6oz dry macaroni
1 garlic clove
4 spring onions
170g/6oz quark skimmed
milk soft cheese
4 tbsp very low-fat natural
fromage frais
1 tsp mild chilli powder
2 level tbsp freshly grated
Parmesan cheese
2 tbsp freshly chopped
chives

1. Preheat the grill to a medium/hot setting. Halve and de-seed the peppers, leaving the stalks intact. Arrange side by side in the grill pan and cook for 7-8 minutes on each side until tender and lightly charred.

2. Meanwhile, bring a saucepan of lightly salted water to the boil and cook the macaroni as directed on the packet – approximately 10-12 minutes. Drain well and return to the saucepan.

3. Peel and crush the garlic. Trim and finely chop the white and green parts of the spring onions. Mix both into the quark and fromage frais. Add the chilli powder and season well.

4. When the macaroni is drained, toss the quark mixture into the pasta and mix well. Pile into each pepper half and press down lightly to fill them properly.

5. Return the peppers to the grill pan and sprinkle with the Parmesan cheese. Place under the grill for a further 3-4 minutes until golden and hot. Serve sprinkled with chopped chives.

mushroom cannelloni

You don't have to eat meat in a cannelloni; an assortment of mushrooms, such as those listed below, makes a delicious, meat-free alternative.

Serves: 4

Preparation and cooking time: approximately 1 hour 30 minutes

454g/1lb assorted mushrooms, eg chestnut, button, shiitake or open cup
1 medium onion
1 garlic clove
1 tbsp freshly chopped thyme or 1 tsp dried
½ tsp ground nutmeg
6 tbsp dry white wine
6 level tbsp couscous, unsoaked
Salt and freshly ground black pepper
200g/7oz can chopped plum tomatoes
700g/1lb 8oz jar passata
2 tsp granulated artificial sweetener
20 dried 'quick-cook' cannelloni tubes
A few sprigs of fresh thyme (optional)
28g/1oz Parmesan cheese

1. Preheat the oven to 200°C/400°F/Gas 6. Wipe and finely chop the mushrooms and place in a saucepan. Peel and finely chop the onion and garlic and add to the mushrooms with thyme, nutmeg and wine. Bring to the boil, cover and simmer for 10 minutes. Stir in the couscous and mix well. Stand for 10 minutes until couscous is tender, season.

2. Meanwhile place the plum tomatoes, passata and sweetener in a blender, blend for a few seconds until smooth and season. Cover the base of an ovenproof dish with a thin layer of sauce.

3. Using the end of a teaspoon, pack each cannelloni tube with the mushroom stuffing. Pile into the dish and pour over the remaining sauce. Top with the thyme sprigs, if using. Cover with foil and bake for 30 minutes. Remove foil and bake for a further 10 minutes or until tender. Remove the thyme and set aside.

4. Preheat the grill to a medium setting. Using a vegetable peeler, shave a few pieces of Parmesan cheese over the cannelloni. Cook for 2-3 minutes until lightly golden and bubbling. Shave over remaining Parmesan cheese, garnish with reserved thyme sprigs, if liked, and serve.

pasta timbales

These pasta moulds make an impressive and attractive course to serve when entertaining. The spinach sauce can be replaced with a simple tomato sauce made from heated passata or chopped canned tomatoes.

Serves: 4
Preparation time: approximately
15 minutes
Cooking time: approximately
35 minutes

Fry Light
1 ripe medium tomato
170g/6oz tricolore spaghetti
Salt and freshly ground
black pepper
1 garlic clove
227g/8oz quark skimmed
milk soft cheese
113g/4oz frozen diced mixed
vegetables, thawed
4 tbsp freshly grated
Parmesan cheese
2 tbsp freshly chopped
chives
2 medium eggs, beaten
340g/12oz frozen chopped
spinach, thawed and drained
142ml/¼pt vegetable stock
¼ tsp ground nutmeg
113g/4oz very low-fat
natural fromage frais

1. Preheat the oven to 220°C/425°F/Gas 7. Lightly spray 4 x 170ml/6fl oz pudding moulds or ramekins with Fry Light. Cut a disc of baking parchment to fit the base of each and press into the bottom. Thinly slice the tomato and arrange on the paper.

2. Break the spaghetti into 5cm/2in lengths. Bring a saucepan of lightly salted water to the boil and cook the spaghetti for 5-6 minutes until just tender. Drain well and place in a mixing bowl.

3. Peel and crush the garlic and mix into the spaghetti along with the quark, mixed vegetables, Parmesan cheese, chives, eggs and plenty of seasoning. Mix well and then pack into the moulds, smoothing off the tops. Bake in the oven for 20-25 minutes until golden and firm. Leave to stand for 10 minutes.

4. Meanwhile, place the spinach in a saucepan along with the stock, nutmeg and seasoning. Bring to the boil, cover and simmer gently for 3 minutes until wilted. Cool for 5 minutes then transfer to a blender or food processor and add the fromage frais. Blend for a few seconds until smooth.

5. Loosen round the edges of the moulds using a pallet knife and turn on to warmed serving plates. Heat the spinach sauce gently without boiling and serve with the pasta moulds.

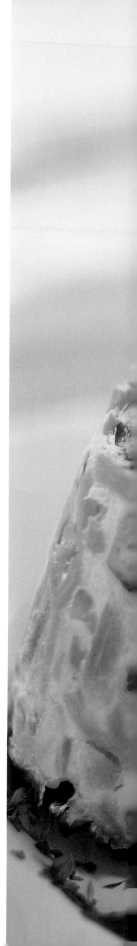

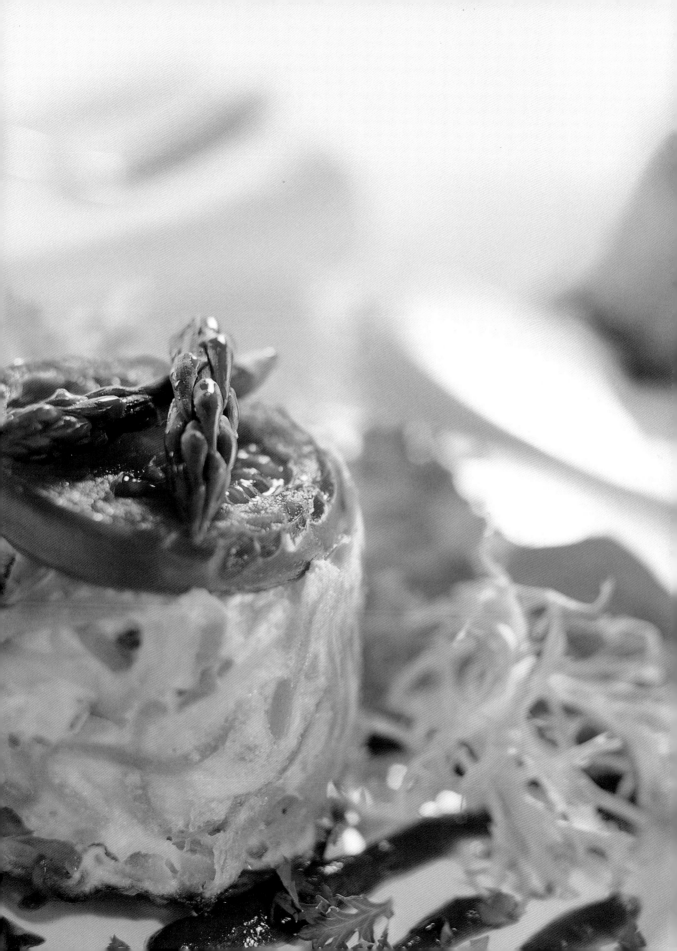

noodles with shredded ginger vegetables

This brilliant one-pot dish not only saves on washing-up, but only takes 30 minutes to prepare and cook. You'll need a lot of cooking space for all these ingredients, so a wok is ideal.

Serves: 4
Preparation and cooking time:
approximately 30 minutes

454g/1lb celeriac
2 large carrots
2 large leeks
1 bunch spring onions
1 garlic clove
5cm/2in piece root ginger
1 tbsp vegetable oil
4 tbsp light soy sauce
250g/9oz bag dried egg
thread noodles
Small bunch fresh chives

1. Prepare the vegetables. Peel the celeriac and carrots and either coarsely grate or cut into thin shreds.

2. Trim the leeks, and slice down the centre. Run under cold water to flush out any trapped earth. Shake well to remove excess water and then shred finely.

3. Trim and chop the spring onions. Peel and finely chop the garlic. Peel and grate or finely shred the ginger.

4. Heat the oil in a large non-stick wok or deep frying pan. Add all the prepared vegetables, and cook over a medium/high heat, stirring, for 4-5 minutes, until well mixed and just starting to soften. Then add the soy sauce and stir-fry for a further 4-5 minutes or until cooked to your liking.

5. Meanwhile, soak or cook the noodles according to the instructions on the packet. Drain well and toss into the cooked vegetables. Mix well, then pile into serving bowls and garnish with the chives.

Cook's Note
If you can't find celeriac in your supermarket, add an extra carrot and two stalks of celery, trimmed and cut into thin strips.

pasta with special pesto

Don't think you have to miss out on your favourite Italian food when losing weight. We've given a low-fat twist to this classic dish, which is packed with the authentic flavour of Italy.

Serves: 4
Preparation and cooking time:
approximately 20 minutes

4 large garlic cloves
14g/½oz fresh basil
170g/6oz quark soft cheese
2 level tbsp freshly grated
Parmesan cheese
salt and freshly ground black
pepper
340g/12oz dried spaghetti
4 plum tomatoes
A few small basil leaves to
garnish

1. To make the pesto: peel and roughly chop the garlic. Place it in a food processor with the basil, quark and Parmesan cheese. Blend for a few seconds until smooth, then season to taste and chill until required.

2. Bring a large saucepan of lightly salted water to the boil and cook the spaghetti according to instructions on the packet. Drain the spaghetti well and return to the pan.

3. Meanwhile, prick the tomatoes, place them in a heatproof bowl and pour over enough boiling water to cover. Leave them for 2 minutes then drain and peel off the skins. Halve the tomatoes, remove the flesh. Set aside.

4. Toss the pesto sauce into the pasta and mix together until spaghetti is well coated. Pile into four warm serving bowls and top with a few pieces of chopped tomato and some small basil leaves. Season with more black pepper if you wish.

vegetable lasagne

When you are in the mood to cook up a treat, follow these four easy steps to create a classic Italian lasagne with a vegetarian twist.

Serves: 4
Preparation and cooking time:
approximately 1 hour

2 medium red onions
1 garlic clove
1 medium red pepper
1 medium orange pepper
1 medium aubergine
1 medium courgettes
2 x 397g/14oz cans chopped
tomatoes with herbs
Salt and freshly ground
black pepper
2 level tbsp tomato purée
2 level tbsp cornflour
284ml/½pt skimmed milk
142ml/¼pt very low-fat
natural fromage frais
6 no-pre-cook lasagne
sheets
4 level tbsp freshly grated
Parmesan cheese

1. Preheat the oven to 200°C/400°F/Gas 6. For the vegetable sauce, peel and finely chop the onions and garlic. Wash and de-seed the peppers. Dice the red pepper and cut the orange pepper into thin strips. Wash and trim the aubergine and courgettes. Dice the aubergine and thinly slice the courgettes.

2. Place the onion, garlic and peppers in a large pan, stir in the canned tomatoes and season. Mix well, bring to the boil, cover and simmer for 10 minutes, stirring after 5 minutes. Add the aubergine and courgettes and cook, uncovered, for 10 minutes, stirring occasionally. Stir in the tomato purée.

3. Meanwhile, make the white sauce. Blend the cornflour with a little of the milk. Pour the remaining milk into a pan, bring to the boil, then add the cornflour mixture, stirring, and cook for 1-2 minutes until thick. Remove from the heat and gradually beat in the fromage frais. Season well.

4. Spoon half the vegetable sauce into an ovenproof baking dish. Lay three lasagne sheets on top, and spread with the remaining vegetable sauce. Top with the remaining lasagne and spread with white sauce. Sprinkle with cheese and bake in the oven for 25-30 minutes until golden and tender.

curried lentil and quorn burgers

Quorn makes a delicious burger and is a great vegetarian alternative when barbecuing. You can vary the flavourings by using different spices such as cumin, coriander and turmeric.

Serves: 4
Preparation and cooking time:
approximately 20 minutes
plus chilling

1 medium onion
small bunch fresh coriander
425g/15oz can green lentils,
drained and rinsed
1 tbsp mild curry powder
salt and freshly ground black
pepper
113g/4oz carrots
113g/4oz Quorn mince

1. Peel the onion and place in a food processor with the coriander, lentils, curry powder and seasoning. Blend for a few seconds until lightly textured. Transfer to a mixing bowl.

2. Peel and finely grate the carrot, and add to the lentil mixture together with the Quorn mince.

3. Divide the mixture into four equal portions and, with wet hands, press into burger shapes approximately 2.5cm/1in thick. Gently transfer to a plate lined with baking parchment and chill for 30 minutes. Note: these burgers do have a crumbly texture.

4. Carefully place the burgers in a wire barbecue basket and place over medium/hot coals to cook for 4-5 minutes on each side until browned and cooked through. Alternatively, place on a grill rack under a preheated medium/hot grill and cook for 5 minutes on each side until golden brown.

Cook's Note
To prevent the mixture sticking to the wire mesh or rack, you may need to brush the wire with a little vegetable oil before placing the burgers inside the basket or on the rack. Look out for non-stick wire barbecue baskets.

pastitso

Based on a classic Greek dish, this recipe is traditionally made with minced lamb. But here, quorn mince makes an excellent substitute. You'll need a large baking dish for this one, so it's ideal to serve when you've got guests for supper.

Serves: 6

Preparation time: approximately 10 minutes plus standing

Cooking time: approximately 1 hour 15 minutes

1 medium onion
1 garlic clove
426ml/¾pt vegetable stock
1 tsp dried oregano
1 tsp ground cinnamon
454g/1lb Quorn mince
397g/14oz can chopped tomatoes
Salt and freshly ground black pepper
227g/8oz macaroni or other similar pasta
340g/12oz very low-fat natural fromage frais
2 medium eggs, beaten
4 level tbsp freshly grated Parmesan cheese

1. Preheat the oven to 180°C/350°F/Gas 4. Peel and finely chop the onion and garlic and place in a saucepan along with 142ml/¼pt of the stock. Bring to the boil, cover and simmer for 5 minutes.

2. Stir in the oregano, cinnamon, Quorn mince, tomatoes and remaining stock. Bring to the boil, cover and simmer for a further 5 minutes. Season well.

3. Meanwhile, bring a saucepan of lightly salted water to the boil and cook the macaroni for 10-12 minutes until just tender. Drain well and mix into the Quorn mince. Pile into an ovenproof dish and place on a baking sheet.

4. Mix the fromage frais with the eggs and some seasoning and spoon over the top of the Quorn and macaroni. Sprinkle with the Parmesan cheese and bake for 50 minutes until the topping is set and lightly golden. Stand for 10 minutes before serving accompanied by a crisp salad.

baked couscous pudding
with chunky chilli vegetable sauce

Depending on how finely you chop the vegetables for this dish will make the sauce chunky or less so. If you prefer a smooth sauce, then blend the vegetables in a food processor and thin it down with more stock if necessary.

Serves: 4
Preparation time: approximately
15 minutes plus soaking
and standing
Cooking time: approximately
45 minutes

227g/8oz pre-cooked
couscous
4 medium eggs, beaten
227g/8oz very low-fat
natural fromage frais
2 tbsp freshly chopped
chives
Salt and freshly ground
black pepper
1 large courgette
2 baby aubergines
142ml/¼pt vegetable stock
397g/14oz can chopped
tomatoes with garlic
½-1 tsp hot chilli powder
Fresh chives to garnish

1. Preheat the oven to 180°C/350°F/Gas 4. Soak the couscous according to the directions on the packet, and then place in a mixing bowl.

2. Stir in the eggs, fromage frais, chives and plenty of seasoning. Mix well and transfer to a small non-stick baking tin lined with baking parchment. Press down well and bake in the oven for 25-30 minutes until firm and lightly crusted. Stand for 10 minutes.

3. Meanwhile make the sauce. Trim and finely dice the courgette and aubergines and place in a saucepan with the stock. Bring to the boil, cover and simmer for 5 minutes. Stir in the tomatoes, chilli powder to taste and seasoning. Bring back to the boil and simmer for a further 5 minutes until thick and tender.

4. Cut the couscous into wedges and serve with the sauce, garnished with fresh chives and sprinkled with more ground black pepper if liked.

chilli quorn, sweetcorn and pepper kebabs

The succulent kebabs can be served hot or cold – either way they are equally delicious. For a special party when you want to impress your guests, you could thread the ingredients on to thick fresh rosemary stems. Just remove most of the green so that only a sprig is left at the end and then push the woody point through the Quorn and vegetables.

Serves: 4
Preparation and cooking time:
approximately 20 minutes

3 corn-on-the-cob
1 small red pepper
1 small green pepper
1 small orange pepper
113g/4oz large Quorn pieces
4 tbsp passata or sieved tomatoes
2 tbsp Worcestershire sauce
½-1 tbsp chilli powder

1. Strip away the leaves and strings from the sweetcorn cobs. Using a large heavy knife, carefully cut each cob into four equal slices. Set aside.

2. Wash the peppers. Halve and de-seed and then cut into 2.5cm/1in cubes. Thread the corn, peppers and Quorn pieces (thread two pieces quorn together) on to four long skewers. Mix together the remaining ingredients and brush over the kebabs.

3. Place the kebabs over hot coals and cook, turning frequently and brushing with the tomato mixture for 7-8 minutes, until tender. Alternatively, place on a grill rack under a preheated hot grill and cook for 7-8 minutes, turning and basting.

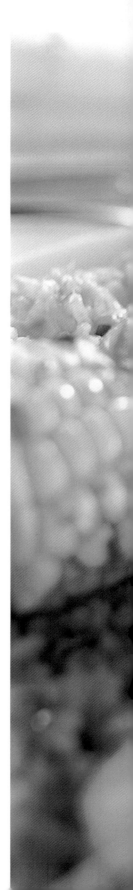

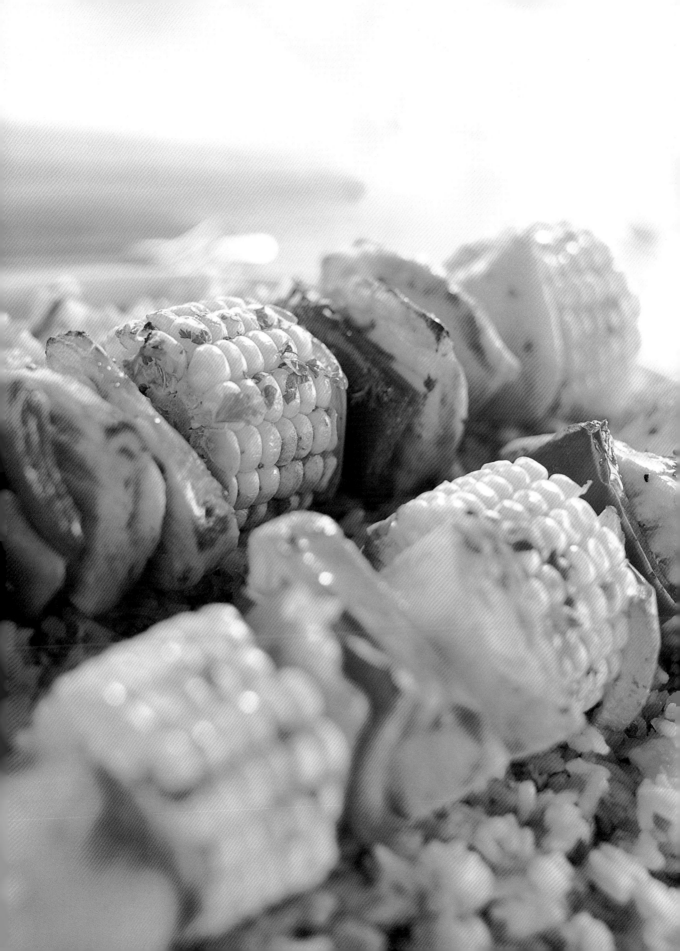

indian-style rice and split peas

Cooking rice with red lentils is very traditional in India and the Middle East. All the flavoured cooking liquid is absorbed during cooking, so the rice is full of spice and taste.

Serves: 4
Preparation time: approximately
15 minutes
Cooking time: approximately
35 minutes

227g/8oz dry basmati rice
113g/4oz raw red lentils
2 bay leaves
2 level tbsp tomato purée
1 tbsp mild curry powder
Salt and freshly ground
black pepper
2 medium onions
¼ cucumber
1 large mild green chilli
4 tbsp freshly chopped
coriander
Fry Light

1. Rinse the rice and lentils under cold running water until it runs clear. Shake well to drain and then place in a large saucepan. Pour over 568ml/1pt water and add the bay leaves, tomato purée, curry powder and seasoning. Bring to the boil, cover and simmer on a very gentle heat for 25-30 minutes until all the liquid has absorbed and the rice and lentils are tender.

2. Meanwhile, peel the onions and slice into 1cm/½in thick slices and separate into rings.

3. Take four of the smaller rings and chop finely. Finely chop the cucumber. Halve and de-seed the chilli and chop this finely. Mix the onion, cucumber and chilli together along with half the coriander and season well. Cover the relish and chill until required.

4. Spray a non-stick frying pan lightly with Fry Light and heat until hot. Add the remaining onion rings and cook for 2-3 minutes on each side until tender and golden. Drain well and keep warm.

5. To serve, discard the bay leaves from the rice and lentils and pile on to four serving plates. Top each with a few onion rings and sprinkle with the remaining chopped coriander. Serve with the cucumber and chilli relish.

mexican green rice

Another one-pot dish that saves on washing up. Experiment with the amount of chilli used: use sparingly at first until you find the amount that suits you best.

Serves: 4
Make and cook: approximately
30 minutes

340g/12oz long grain white rice
1.2 litres/2pt vegetable stock made with Vecon
Salt and freshly ground black pepper
1 tbsp ground coriander
1 large onion
2 large green peppers
2 fresh mild green chillies
2 medium courgettes
227g/8oz frozen peas
4 tbsp freshly chopped coriander

1. Place the rice in a large saucepan and pour over the stock. Season well and add the ground coriander. Bring the stock to the boil, cover and simmer for 10 minutes.

2. Meanwhile, prepare the vegetables. Peel and finely chop the onion. Halve, de-seed and slice the peppers into thin strips. Halve, de-seed and chop the chillies. Trim and dice the courgettes.

3. Stir in the prepared vegetables, bring back to the boil, cover and simmer for 5 minutes – if the mixture becomes too dry, then add some more liquid.

4. Stir in the frozen peas, and continue to cook, uncovered, for a further 4-5 minutes until tender and the stock has been absorbed.

5. Taste and adjust the seasoning if necessary. Stir in the chopped coriander and serve immediately, accompanied by a crisp salad.

Cook's Notes
Take care when preparing chillies as their juices can irritate the skin. Avoid touching your eyes. Always rinse your hands in cold water after preparation or wear thin gloves.

Add fibre to this dish by using brown rice instead of white: if you do, increase cooking time in step 1 by 15 minutes.

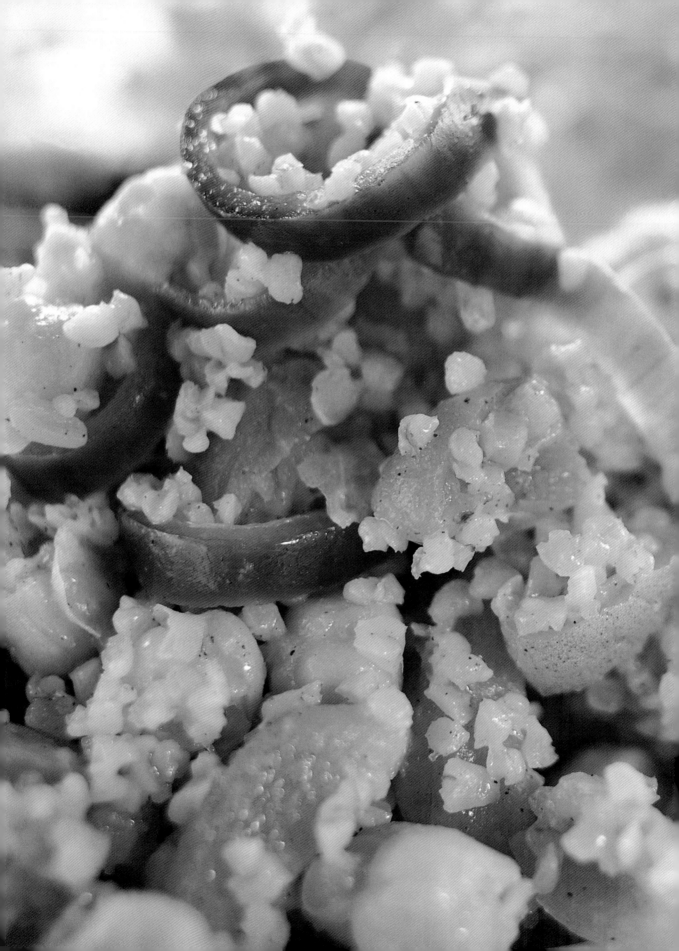

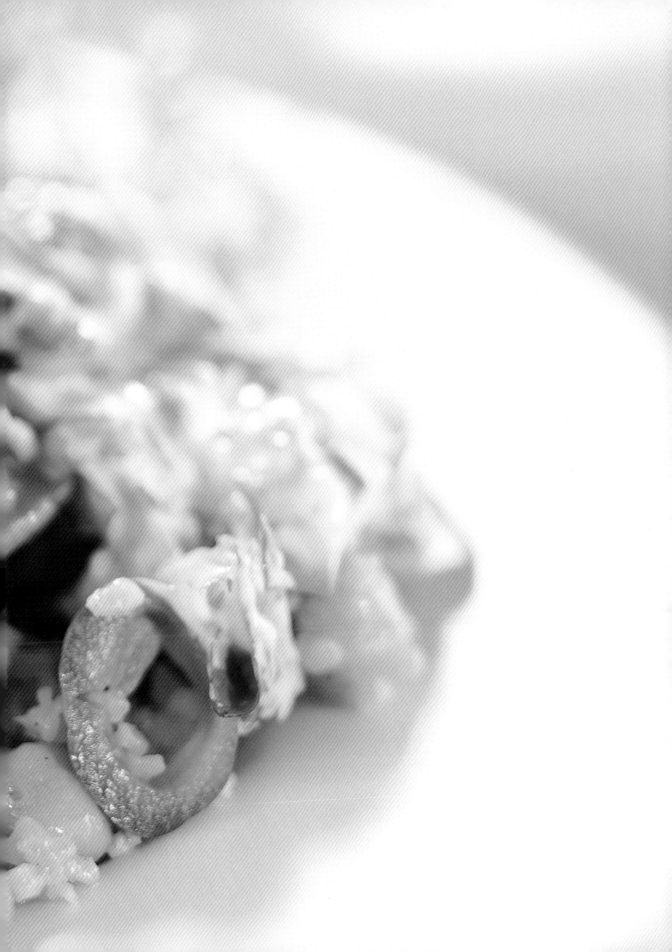

pumpkin risotto

This brightly coloured dish of golden-orange pumpkin, red onion and white rice makes a substantial supper for four or a classic Italian starter for six. Omit the blue cheese if preferred.

Serves: 4
Preparation time: approximately
15 minutes
Cooking time: approximately
50 minutes

454g/1lb pumpkin or squash
1 large red onion
1 tbsp lemon juice
852ml/1½pt vegetable stock
1 garlic clove
340g/12oz dry arborio rice
A pinch of saffron
Salt and freshly ground
black pepper
28g/1oz piece Stilton blue
cheese
2 tbsp freshly chopped
parsley

1. Slice the skin from the pumpkin and discard the seeds. Cut into 2cm/¾in chunks. Peel and finely slice the onion and toss in the lemon juice. Transfer both vegetables to a saucepan and pour over 284ml/½pt stock. Bring to the boil, cover and simmer for about 15 minutes until just tender. Turn off the heat and keep covered.

2. Peel and finely chop the garlic and place in a saucepan with the rice and 284ml/½pt stock. Bring to the boil and simmer for 5 minutes until the stock has almost evaporated.

3. Meanwhile, heat the remaining stock until just about to boil, and reduce the heat to maintain the temperature. Add the saffron and seasoning to the rice mixture and add a ladleful of stock; cook gently, stirring until absorbed.

4. Continue ladling in the stock until the liquid is absorbed and the rice is thick, creamy and tender. Keep the heat moderate. This will take 20-25 minutes.

5. Drain the pumpkin and red onion and stir gently into the rice. Heat through for 2 minutes.

6. Ladle into warmed serving bowls and crumble a little blue cheese on to each. Sprinkle with black pepper and parsley to serve.

spicy tabbouleh with apricots

This Middle Eastern-style dish is usually laced with olive oil, but this healthier version is so packed full with the rich flavours of lemon juice, cinnamon and dried apricots that you won't miss it at all.

Serves: 4
Preparation time: approximately
12 minutes plus standing
Cooking time: approximately
12 minutes

I large red onion
I tbsp lemon juice
227g/8oz bulgur wheat
852ml/1½pt vegetable stock
113g/4oz no-need-to-soak
dried apricots
397g/14oz can chickpeas,
drained and rinsed
I tsp ground cinnamon
Salt and freshly ground
black pepper
¼ cucumber
15g/½oz pack fresh
coriander
113g/4oz very low-fat
natural yogurt

1. Peel and finely slice the onion and toss in the lemon juice. Place in a large saucepan along with the bulgur wheat and stock. Bring to the boil, cover and simmer for 10 minutes.

2. Meanwhile, finely slice the apricots. Stir into the bulgur wheat along with the chickpeas, cinnamon and plenty of seasoning. Cover, remove from the heat and leave to stand for 10 minutes until all the stock has been absorbed.

3. Meanwhile, finely chop the cucumber and coriander. Serve the tabbouleh with the cucumber, coriander and yogurt on top.

Cook's Note
You can allow this dish to cool completely and then chill. It is delicious served as a salad.

Illustrated on previous page

cassoulet

This French bean stew is good served with mashed potato, rice or pasta as a hearty meal on a cold day. Using canned beans cuts down the preparation and cooking time.

Serves: 4
Preparation time: approximately 10 minutes
Cooking time: approximately 20 minutes

1 medium onion
1 garlic clove
142ml/¼pt vegetable stock
1 tsp dried mixed herbs
2 bay leaves
2 x 425g/15oz cans mixed pulses, drained and rinsed
142ml/¼pt dry red wine
426ml/¾pt passata
227g/8oz Quorn pieces
Salt and freshly ground black pepper
2 tbsp freshly chopped parsley

1. Peel and finely chop the onion and garlic. Place in a large saucepan along with the stock. Bring to the boil, cover and simmer for 5 minutes.

2. Stir in the dried herbs, bay leaves, pulses, wine and passata. Bring to the boil, cover and simmer for 10 minutes. Stir in the Quorn pieces and plenty of seasoning, and simmer, uncovered, for a further 5 minutes. Discard the bay leaves.

3. Serve sprinkled with chopped parsley and accompanied by green vegetables.

mushroom stroganoff

A mildly flavoured stew of meaty mushrooms cooked in a tomato sauce. Traditionally, the yogurt is stirred into the sauce, but here you should spoon it over just before serving to prevent curdling and spoiling the appearance.

Serves: 4
Preparation time: approximately
10 minutes
Cooking time: approximately
15 minutes

227g/8oz shallots or baby onions
426ml/¾pt vegetable stock
227g/8oz baby button mushrooms
225g/8oz assorted larger mushrooms such as open cup, chestnut and shiitake
2 level tbsp tomato purée
½ tsp ground nutmeg
Salt and freshly ground black pepper
113g/4oz very low-fat natural yogurt
1 tsp caraway seeds (optional)
2 tbsp freshly chopped parsley

1. Peel and halve the shallots or onions. Place in a large saucepan and add 142ml/¼pt of the stock. Bring to the boil, cover and simmer for 5 minutes.

2. Wipe all the mushrooms, and halve the larger ones. Blend the remaining stock with the tomato purée. Pour into the saucepan along with the mushrooms, nutmeg and plenty of seasoning. Bring to the boil, cover and simmer for 10 minutes until tender.

3. Serve each portion with a spoonful of yogurt on top, sprinkled with caraway seeds, if using, and chopped parsley.

root vegetable and lentil casserole

A hearty, satisfying combination of comforting vegetables cooked in a mildly spicy stock, thickened with red lentils. Serve simply with green vegetables.

Serves: 4
Preparation time: approximately
15 minutes
Cooking time: approximately
40 minutes

1 medium onion
2 celery sticks
852ml/1½pt chicken stock made with Bovril
227g/8oz carrots
227g/8oz potatoes
227g/8oz parsnips
227g/8oz swede
1 large leek
1 tsp paprika
1 tsp ground cumin
1 tsp ground coriander
1 tsp mustard seeds, crushed
Salt and freshly ground black pepper
113g/4oz red lentils
2 tbsp freshly chopped coriander

1. Peel the onion and slice thinly. Trim and slice the celery. Place in a large saucepan with 142ml/¼pt stock. Bring to the boil, cover and simmer for 5 minutes.

2. Meanwhile, peel and slice the carrots. Peel the potatoes, parsnips and swede and cut into small chunks. Trim and slice the leek lengthwise and rinse under running water to flush out any trapped earth. Shake well and slice thickly.

3. Stir the vegetables into the saucepan along with the remaining stock, spices, plenty of seasoning and the lentils. Bring to the boil, cover and cook for 30 minutes or until the vegetables are tender.

4. Serve the casserole sprinkled with chopped coriander and accompanied by green vegetables.

beany sausages and tomato sauce

This tasty treat is sure to be a great hit with all the family and with it only taking 30 minutes from start to finish, it's really quick too!

Serves: 4

Preparation and cooking time: approximately 30 minutes

397g/14oz can kidney beans in water, drained
6 spring onions
Salt and freshly ground black pepper
½ tsp mixed dried herbs
142g/5oz carrots
Fry Light

For the tomato sauce:
284ml/½pt passata
1 tbsp malt vinegar
1 tbsp Worcestershire sauce
Dash of Tabasco sauce
½ tsp artificial sweetener

1. Place the beans in a food processor or blender. Trim and roughly chop the spring onions. Add to the beans along with plenty of seasoning and the mixed herbs. Blend for a few seconds until smooth. Alternatively, mash the beans with a potato masher or fork.

2. Peel and grate the carrots and stir into the mixture. Divide into eight portions and form into sausage shapes about 7cm/3in long.

3. Heat a non-stick frying pan until hot and spray with ten applications of Fry Light. Add the bean sausages and cook, turning frequently, for ten minutes until browned all over.

4. Meanwhile make the tomato sauce. Place the passata, vinegar, Worcestershire sauce, Tabasco sauce, salt and artificial sweetener in a bowl and mix well to form a smooth sauce. Heat for 2-3 minutes, stirring continuously, until hot.

5. Serve two sausages each with mashed potato, green vegetables and tomato sauce, sprinkled with fresh parsley, if desired.

ratatouille with eggs

Here is a combination of sweet Mediterranean vegetables cooked in a pan with eggs broken into the top and cooked whole so that they absorb all the flavours from the sauce.

Serves: 4
Preparation time: approximately
15 minutes
Cooking time: approximately
20 minutes

1 medium onion
1 small red pepper
1 small yellow pepper
1 large courgette
2 baby aubergines
2 x 397g/14oz cans chopped
tomatoes with garlic
1 tsp dried mixed herbs
Salt and freshly ground
black pepper
4 large eggs

1. Peel the onion and slice thinly. Halve and de-seed the peppers and cut into thin strips. Trim and slice the courgette and aubergines.

2. Place all the vegetables in a deep medium-sized non-stick frying pan and mix in the tomatoes, herbs and seasoning. Bring to the boil, stirring, cover and simmer for 10 minutes until the vegetables are just tender.

3. Mix well and spread the vegetables evenly across the frying pan. Make four indents in the mixture and break an egg into each. Cook over a gentle heat for 10 minutes or until the eggs have set.

4. Serve straight from the frying pan with freshly cooked rice and a crisp salad to accompany.

spanish-style tortilla

This thick omelette of potatoes, peppers and onions makes a delicious supper served hot or cold. Simply cut into wedges and serve straight from the pan.

Serves: 4
Preparation time: approximately
15 minutes
Cooking time: approximately
40 minutes

681g/1½lb potatoes
Salt and freshly ground
black pepper
1 large onion
1 garlic clove
1 large red pepper
1 large green pepper
Fry Light
6 large eggs, beaten
2 tbsp freshly chopped
parsley

1. Peel the potatoes and slice very thinly. Place in a large saucepan and cover with water. Add a pinch of salt and bring to the boil, cook for 3 minutes then drain well.

2. Meanwhile, peel and finely chop the onion and garlic and place in a saucepan. Halve and de-seed the peppers. Slice thinly and mix into the onion and garlic. Pour over 284ml/½pt water. Bring to the boil, cover and simmer for 5 minutes. Drain well.

3. Spray a deep medium sized non-stick frying pan with Fry Light and heat until hot. Add the potato slices, peppers and onion. Stir well to mix.

4. Season the eggs and pour into the pan, packing the vegetables firmly together. Lower the heat and cook for 15-20 minutes until set. Carefully loosen and slide on to a plate. Respray the pan and heat until hot. Carefully slide the tortilla back into the pan, the other way up, and cook for a further 10 minutes until tender.

sweetcorn pasta bake

The ultimate comfort food, this pasta bake has a delicious creamy sauce. Small pasta shapes work best in this recipe, but you could use short lengths of spaghetti or tagliatelle as an alternative.

Serves 4
Preparation and cooking time:
approximately 1 hour

227g/8oz small dried pasta shapes
1 bunch spring onions
1 small red pepper
227g/8oz canned sweetcorn kernels, drained
200g/7oz low-fat soft cheese
397g/14oz very low-fat natural fromage frais
2 large eggs, beaten
Salt and freshly ground black pepper
Fresh chives to garnish

1. Preheat the oven to 200°C/400°F/Gas 6. Bring a large saucepan of lightly salted water to the boil and cook the pasta according to the packet instructions. Drain well.

2. Meanwhile, trim and chop the spring onions and halve, de-seed and chop the pepper. Place in a heatproof mixing bowl and stir in the sweetcorn, soft cheese fromage frais and eggs. Beat until well blended.

3. Mix in the drained pasta and add plenty of seasoning. Pile into an ovenproof dish and level off the surface. Sprinkle with grated parmesan cheese if desired. Stand the dish in a roasting tin and pour in sufficient boiling water to come half way up the side of the dish. Bake in the oven for 30-35 minutes until firm and golden.

4. Garnish with fresh chives and serve with a crisp salad.

quorn chilli with
spicy potato wedges

Chilli is a real family favourite and this delicious recipe is bound to go down well. The potato wedges make an ideal accompaniment.

Serves: 4
Preparation and cooking time:
approximately 1 hour

4x 227g/8oz baking potatoes
Fry Light
2 tsp chilli powder
1 medium onion
1 garlic clove
426ml/¾pt beef stock made
with Bovril
454g/1lb Quorn mince
397g/14oz can chopped
tomatoes
425g/15oz can kidney beans
in water, drained and rinsed
Salt and freshly ground
black pepper
2 spring onions
Very low-fat natural
fromage frais to garnish

1. Preheat the oven to 200°C /400°F/ Gas Mark 6. Wash and scrub the baking potatoes and cut them into wedges about 1cm/½in thick. Arrange skin-side down on a baking sheet lined with baking parchment and spray lightly with Fry Light. Sprinkle with 1 tsp of the chilli powder and bake in the oven for 30-35 minutes, turning occasionally until tender and golden.

2. Meanwhile, peel and finely chop the onion and garlic and place in a saucepan along with 142ml/¼pt of the beef stock. Bring to the boil, then reduce the heat, cover and simmer for about 5 minutes.

3. Stir in the Quorn mince, tomatoes, kidney beans and remaining stock. Add sufficient chilli powder to taste and season well. Bring to the boil, cover and simmer for 10 minutes.

4. To serve, trim and chop the spring onions. Drain the potato wedges and serve with the chilli, garnished with a little fromage frais and sprinkled with chopped spring onion and chilli powder.

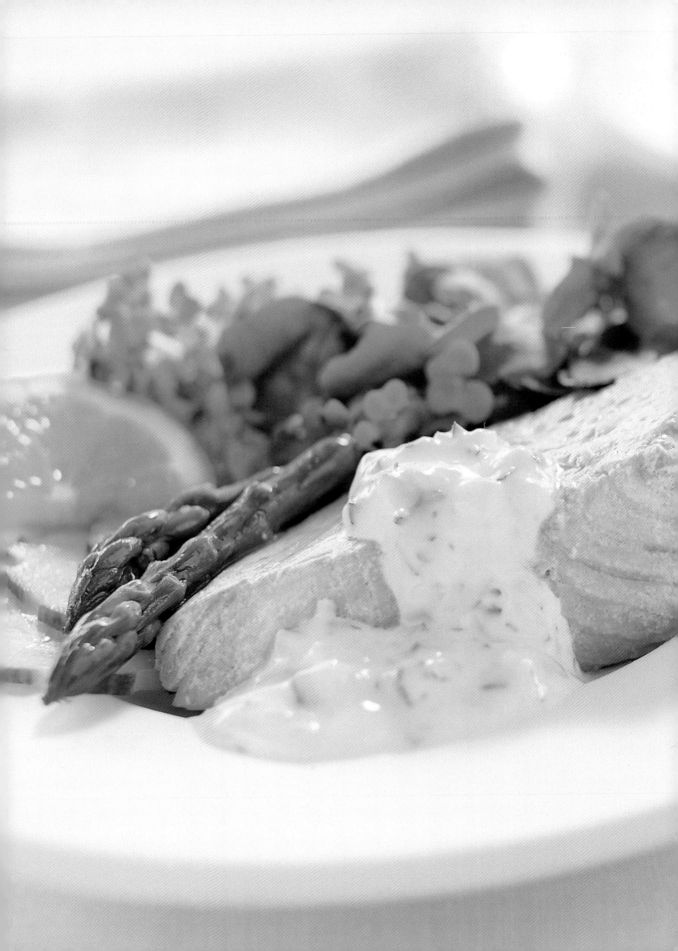

vegetables and salads

fruity coronation chicken

A classic salad usually made with mayonnaise and whipped cream, this version is much lighter and full of Indian flavours. It is also good made with large peeled prawns instead of the chicken.

Serves: 4
Preparation time: approximately
20 minutes

454g/1lb skinless lean cooked chicken meat
4 ripe peaches
4 tbsp very low-fat natural fromage frais
2 tbsp low-calorie mayonnaise
2 tsp mild curry powder
1 level tbsp spicy mango chutney
Salt and freshly ground black pepper
15g/½oz pack fresh coriander
113g/4oz mixed small salad leaves
14g/½oz toasted flaked almonds

1. Cut the chicken into bite-sized pieces and place in a bowl. Wash and dry the peaches, then halve and stone them, and slice into thin wedges.

2. Mix the fromage frais, mayonnaise, curry powder and chutney together and season. Stir into the cooked chicken and peaches until well mixed.

3. Mix half the coriander with the salad leaves and pile on to four serving plates. Top with the chicken and peach mixture and sprinkle with remaining coriander leaves. Lightly crumble the flaked almonds over the top of each portion.

ham and pineapple rolls

These tasty rolls of ham and cheese would make an excellent light lunch, and they could easily be packed into a plastic container for a more portable meal.

Serves: 4
Preparation time: approximately
20 minutes

12 thin large slices lean ham
255g/9oz carton very low-fat
cottage cheese
113g/4oz fresh pineapple
flesh
½ small red pepper
1 stick celery
2 tbsp freshly chopped
chives
Salt and freshly ground
black pepper
113g/4oz mixed salad leaves
Chives to garnish

1. Remove any excess fat from the ham and set aside.

2. Place the cottage cheese in a bowl. Finely chop the pineapple and mix into the cottage cheese. Halve, de-seed and finely chop the pepper. Trim and finely chop the celery. Mix into the cottage cheese along with the chives and seasoning.

3. Divide the filling between the ham slices, and roll each one up.

4. Serve three rolls per person on a bed of a few salad leaves. Garnish with the chives and serve sprinkled with black pepper.

roast beef with mexican-style coleslaw

This is an excellent recipe for using up leftover cooked meat. Alternatively, you can buy ready sliced cooked beef or other meat from the delicatessen or supermarket.

Serves: 4

Preparation time: approximately 20 minutes plus chilling

½ red cabbage
1 small onion
1 small red pepper
113g/4oz radishes
2 tbsp freshly chopped coriander
4 tbsp very low-fat natural fromage frais
2 level tsp chilli sauce
1 lime
Salt and freshly ground black pepper
340g/12oz lean roast beef, thinly sliced
A few coriander leaves to garnish

1. Remove the central stalk from the cabbage and finely shred the leaves. Peel and finely chop the onion. Wash and dry the pepper, then cut in half, de-seed and finely chop. Wash, dry and grate the radishes. Place all the vegetables in a bowl and mix in the chopped coriander.

2. Mix the fromage frais with the chilli sauce. Finely grate the rind from the lime and extract the juice. Mix into the fromage frais. Season well.

3. Stir the chilli dressing into the vegetables and mix well. Cover and chill for 30 minutes.

4. Arrange the beef between four serving plates and spoon on the coleslaw. Serve sprinkled with fresh coriander.

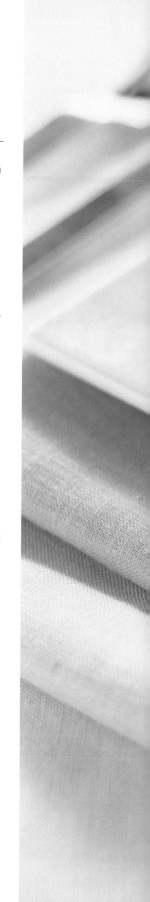

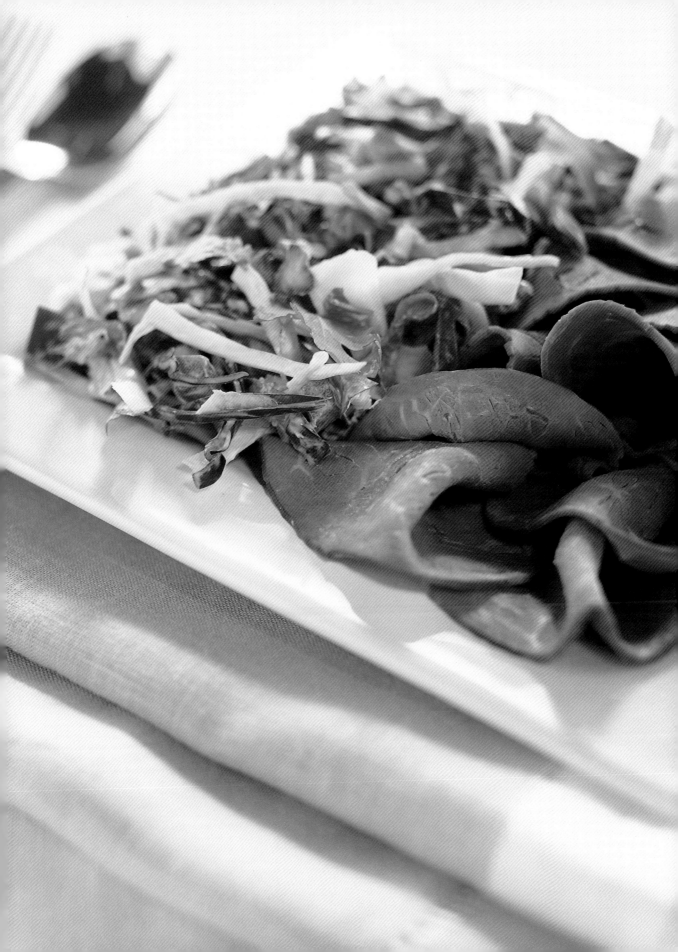

mini-lamb koftas

These mini-lamb koftas are ideal to serve as a starter or as party snacks. This recipe is full of flavour – and with no added fat.

Makes: 15
Preparation and cooking time:
approximately 20 minutes

340g/12oz extra lean minced lamb
1 garlic clove, crushed
1 tsp cinnamon
1 tsp cumin
2 tbsp freshly chopped coriander
Salt and freshly ground pepper
1 medium egg yolk

1. Preheat the oven to 190°C/375°F/Gas 5. In a bowl, mix together the lamb and the rest of the dry ingredients.

2. Bind together with the egg yolk. Then form into 15 balls and place on a baking sheet.

3. Bake in the oven for 15 minutes until cooked through. Drain on kitchen paper and serve warm on cocktail sticks sprinkled with more chopped coriander.

cauliflower and potato curry

This Indian-style dish makes an excellent accompaniment to a plain rice or lentil dish. For a spicier flavour, experiment with a hotter curry spice blend.

Serves: 4
Preparation time: approximately
15 minutes plus standing
Cooking time: approximately
40 minutes

454g/1lb potatoes
227g/8oz carrots
227g/8oz cauliflower
1 medium onion
1 garlic clove
2.5cm/1in piece root ginger
1 fresh green chilli
1 tbsp mild curry powder
1 stick cinnamon, broken
1 bay leaf
14g/½oz block creamed coconut
397g/14oz can chopped tomatoes
Salt and freshly ground black pepper
2 tbsp freshly chopped coriander

1. Peel the potatoes and carrots and cut into small chunks. Break the cauliflower into small florets, and set aside.

2. Peel and roughly chop the onion and garlic. Peel and roughly chop the ginger. Halve and de-seed the chilli, then roughly chop. Place in a blender or food processor and blend until it forms a smooth paste. Place in a large saucepan along with the curry powder, cinnamon stick and bay leaf. Pour in 142ml/¼pt water, bring to the boil, cover and simmer for 5 minutes.

3. Add the vegetables to the saucepan and stir to coat in the spice paste. Grate in the coconut and pour in a further 284ml/½pt water. Add the tomatoes and plenty of seasoning and bring to the boil. Cover and simmer for 30 minutes until tender. Allow to stand for 5 minutes. Discard the bay leaf and cinnamon.

4. Serve sprinkled with chopped coriander.

slimming world's syn-free chips

Chips are high on the list of food that's hard to give up when you are losing weight – and the good news is that with our low-fat version you don't have to!

Serves: 4
Preparation and cooking time:
approximately 40 minutes

908g/2lb medium-sized
Maris Piper potatoes
Fry Light
Crushed sea salt and malt
vinegar (optional)

1. Preheat oven to 240°C/475°F/Gas 9. Peel the potatoes using a potato peeler and remove any blemishes or 'eyes'. Slice lengthwise into approximately 1cm/½in thick rectangular chips.

2. Bring a large saucepan of salted water to the boil. Add the chips and cook for 4 minutes. Drain and leave aside for 10 minutes to dry.

3. Return the chips to the dry saucepan, cover with a lid and shake to 'rough up' the edges of the chips – this 'roughness' is important to the texture of the chips.

4. Spray a metal baking tray with Fry Light. Transfer the chips to the tray, spray lightly with Fry Light and bake in the oven for 20-25 minutes, turning occasionally, until golden brown on all sides. Drain them on absorbent kitchen paper and serve with salt and vinegar.

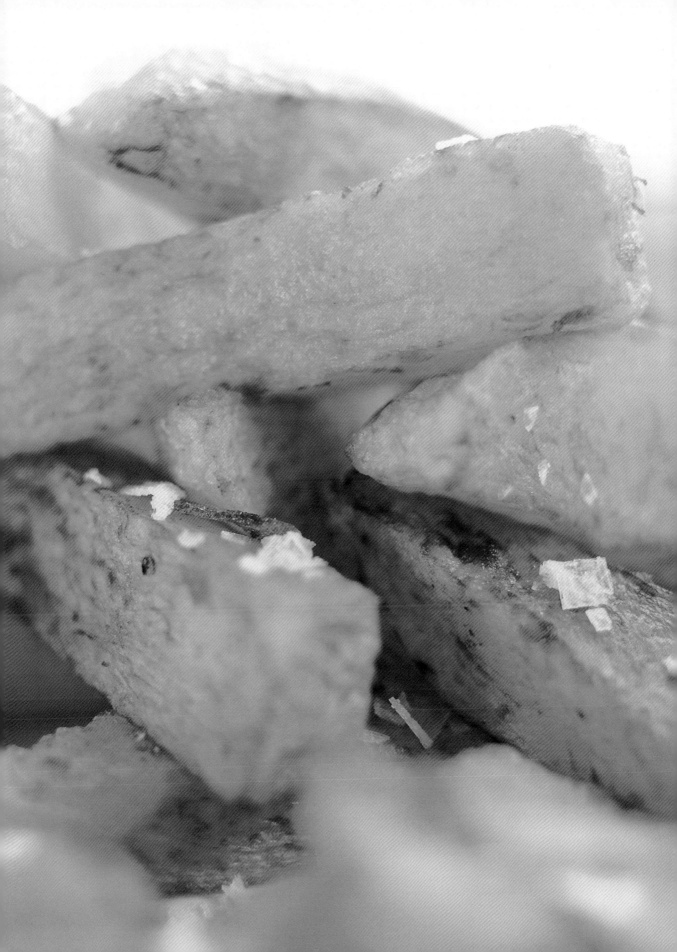

dolmades

Dolmades are another great idea for a delicious low-fat starter, or to serve as nibbles when entertaining friends.

Makes: about 25 servings
Preparation and cooking time:
approximately 40 minutes

1 medium red onion, finely chopped
2 tbsp lemon juice
1 tsp unsweetened mint sauce
227g/8oz cooked white rice
1 tsp ground cumin
Salt and freshly ground black pepper
1 medium egg yolk
25 vine leaves
strips of spring onion, blanched

1. Place the chopped onion in a small saucepan with the lemon juice and simmer for 3-4 minutes, stirring, until softened. Remove from the heat and stir in the mint sauce, cooked white rice, ground cumin and plenty of seasoning. Bind together with the egg yolk.

2. Prepare 25 vine leaves as directed on the packet. Drain well and dry using absorbent kitchen paper.

3. Lay each vine leaf, vein side up, on a board. Place a spoonful of rice in the middle. Fold in two parallel sides of the leaf and roll up the leaf to encase the stuffing completely.

4. Place in a steaming compartment or colander over a pan of boiling water. Cover and steam for 10 minutes until hot. Drain and serve warm, tied in blanched strips of spring onion.

garlic and rosemary roast baby potatoes

Here is a delicious way to bake potatoes without any fat. Try baking with different herbs like thyme or sage, or add some sliced onion and fennel seeds.

Serves: 4
Preparation time: approximately
10 minutes
Cooking time: approximately
1 hour 10 minutes

908g/2lb baby potatoes
2 garlic cloves
A few sprigs rosemary
4 tbsp vegetable stock
Coarse salt and freshly
ground black pepper
Fresh rosemary to garnish

1. Preheat the oven to 200°C/400°F/Gas 6. Scrub the potatoes and place in a large ovenproof casserole. Peel the garlic and slice thinly. Push in amongst the potatoes along with sprigs of rosemary.

2. Spoon over the stock, cover with a sheet of foil and place the lid on top. Bake in the oven for about an hour or until tender.

3. Increase the oven temperature to 230°C/450°F/Gas 8. Transfer the potatoes to a non-stick baking tray using a draining spoon. Season with coarse salt and black pepper. Bake for a further 10 minutes until lightly golden. Discard the baked rosemary and replace with fresh rosemary to garnish.

spicy red roast vegetables

This spicy sauce is an excellent way to liven up vegetables. The soy sauce and passata give the vegetables a rich, browny-red colour together with a deliciously savoury flavour.

Serves: 4
Preparation time: approximately
20 minutes
Cooking time: approximately
40 minutes

1 medium red pepper
1 medium yellow pepper
8 shallots or baby onions
1 large courgette
1 bulb fennel
113g/4oz baby corn
170g/6oz large chestnut or
large closed cup mushrooms
1 garlic clove
3 tbsp dark soy sauce
3 tbsp passata
1 tsp Chinese five spice
powder
½-1 tsp hot chilli powder
1 level tbsp clear honey

1. Preheat the oven to 220°C/425°F/Gas 7. Halve and de-seed the peppers, and cut each half in half again. Peel the shallots or baby onions. Trim the courgette and cut diagonally into 1cm/½in thick slices. Trim and quarter the fennel lengthwise. Trim the baby corn. Wipe the mushrooms. Peel and crush the garlic.

2. Place the peppers, onions, fennel and garlic in a large bowl. Mix the soy sauce, passata, five spice powder, chilli powder and honey together and toss into the vegetables.

3. Transfer the vegetables to a large shallow non-stick baking sheet using a draining spoon. Bake in the oven for 20 minutes, turning and basting occasionally.

4. Meanwhile, toss the courgette, mushrooms and baby corn in the remaining sauce and mix into the other vegetables. Cook for a further 15-20 minutes until the vegetables are rich brown and tender. Serve immediately.

Cook's Note
You won't need to season these vegetables as soy sauce is salty enough.

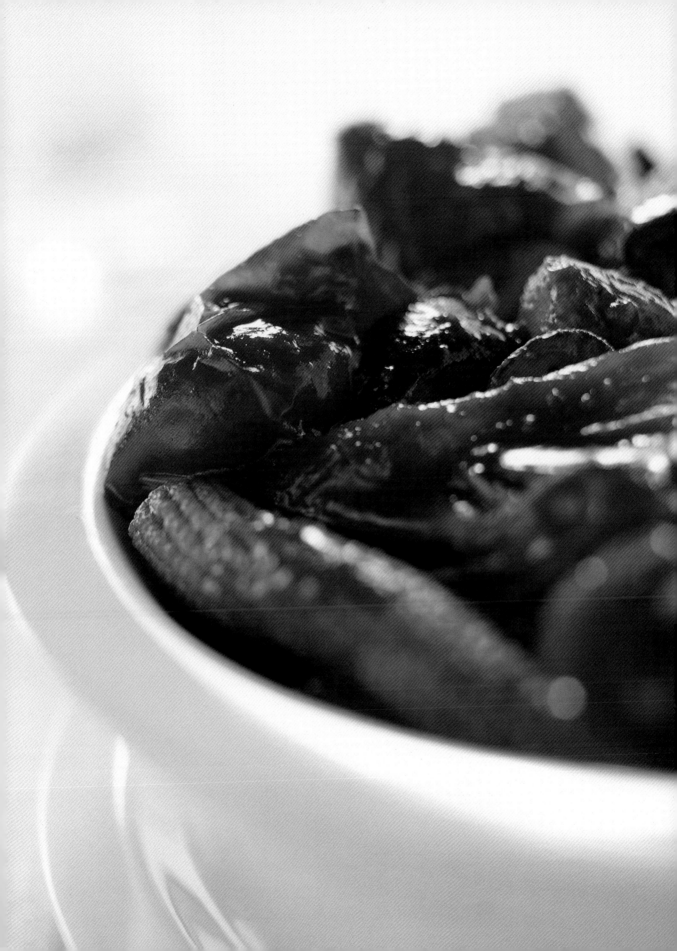

maple baked roots

For this recipe, make sure you cut the vegetables to an even size so that they cook evenly. Although they take a while to cook, this dish is full of flavour and requires no fat.

Serves: 4
Preparation time: approximately
15 minutes
Cooking time: approximately
1 hour 30 minutes

227g/8oz baby parsnips
227g/8oz small carrots
227g/8oz small roasting
potatoes, such as King
Edwards, about the size of
eggs
227g/8oz swede
A few bay leaves
Juice of 1 lemon
4 level tbsp maple syrup
Coarse salt and freshly
ground black pepper

1. Preheat the oven to 200°C/400°F/Gas 6. Peel the baby parsnips and carrots, halve lengthwise and place in the bottom of a large ovenproof casserole with a lid.

2. Peel the potatoes and cut in half. Peel the swede and cut into chunks about the same size as the potatoes. Place in the casserole and mix well. Push the bay leaves in amongst the vegetables.

3. Mix the lemon juice and maple syrup together and pour over the vegetables. Season well. Cover the casserole with a sheet of foil and then place the lid on top. Bake in the oven for about 1½ hours or until tender and cooked through. Drain and discard the bay leaves. Serve seasoned with coarse salt and black pepper.

Cook's Notes
You can use sweet potatoes in this recipe, but you will need to parboil them whole and unpeeled for 20-30 minutes, depending on their size, until just tender. Drain, cool and peel. Cut into 2.5cm/1in thick wedges and add to the casserole.

Turnip would work well too – simply prepare as for swede.

mustard baked potato wedges

Try these baked potatoes with a twist. They can be served to accompany a main course or make a delicious snack by themselves.

Makes: about 30
Preparation and cooking time:
approximately 40 minutes

2 x 227g/8oz baking
potatoes
1 tbsp vegetable oil
2 tsp dry mustard powder
2 tsp paprika
½ tsp cayenne pepper
2 tsp coarse sea salt

1. Preheat the oven to 200°C/400°F/Gas 6. Scrub the baking potatoes and cut into 1cm/½in thick wedges.

2. Place the wedges in a large clean plastic bag and add the vegetable oil, dry mustard powder, paprika and cayenne pepper. Seal and shake well to mix.

3. Arrange them, skin side down, on a lined baking sheet, sprinkle with the coarse sea salt and bake for 30-35 minutes, turning occasionally, until tender and lightly golden. Drain and serve hot.

stir-fried summer vegetables

An alternative to a traditional Oriental stir-fry, which makes the most of the delicate flavours of some our most tasty vegetables.

Serves: 4
Preparation time: approximately
15 minutes
Cooking time: approximately
10 minutes

85g/3oz sugar snap peas
85g/3oz baby carrots
85g/3oz thin green beans
85g/3oz fine asparagus
spears
1 medium leek
Fry Light
2 tbsp unsweetened orange
juice
2 tbsp light soy sauce
2 level tsp clear honey
85g/3oz beansprouts
½ tsp finely grated orange
zest
1 tbsp freshly chopped
chives

1. Trim the sugar snap peas. Scrub and trim the baby carrots. Top the green beans. Cut the woody ends from the asparagus. Trim the leek and slice lengthwise. Rinse under cold running water to remove any trapped earth, then shred finely.

2. Spray a non-stick wok or large frying pan lightly with Fry Light and heat until hot. Stir-fry the leek for 2 minutes until wilted. Add the carrots, green beans and asparagus along with the orange juice and stir-fry for 3 minutes.

3. Add the sugar snap peas, soy sauce and honey and stir fry for a further 2 minutes. Add the beansprouts and orange rind and stir-fry for a further minute or until the vegetables are cooked to your liking.

4. Serve immediately sprinkled with the chopped chives.

Cook's Note
It is important to keep the vegetables moving in the wok while they are cooking to ensure they cook evenly.

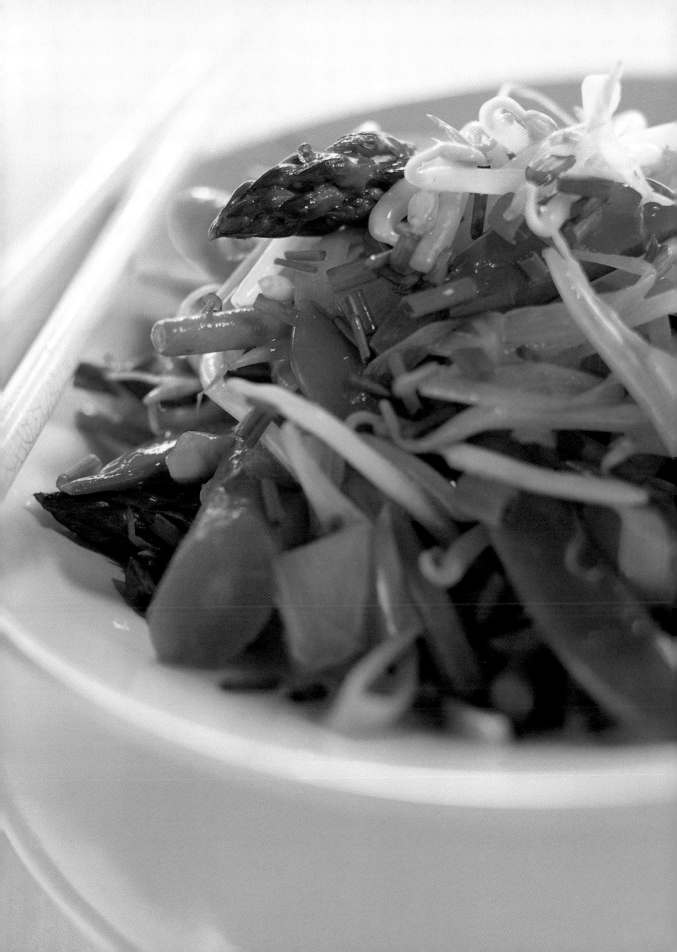

artichoke and cherry tomato salad

Artichokes are an often forgotten vegetable, but they have a subtle flavour and look very attractive as part of a salad platter.

Serves: 4
Preparation time: approximately
15 minutes

227g/8oz cherry tomatoes
2 x 397g/14oz cans
artichoke hearts, drained
and rinsed
1 bunch spring onions
2 stalks of celery with leaves
4 tbsp very low-fat natural
yogurt
2 level tbsp low calorie
mayonnaise
½ tsp finely grated lemon
rind
Pinch of cayenne pepper
¼ tsp celery salt

1. Remove the stalks from the cherry tomatoes and wash and pat dry. Cut them in half and place in a serving bowl.

2. Quarter the artichoke hearts and toss gently into the tomatoes. Trim and slice the white and green parts of the spring onions. Trim, wash and chop the stalks and leaves of the celery. Sprinkle over the salad, and lightly mix in.

3. Mix the remaining ingredients together and serve as a dressing to accompany the salad.

Cook's Notes
Spring onions give a rich, strong, oniony flavour. For a milder flavour you can use freshly chopped chives or a shredded raw leek instead.

If preferred, you can toss the dressing into the salad before serving.

chinese vegetable salad

Crisp, colourful vegetables add the texture to this flavoured tofu dish. It sounds unusual, but it is very tasty, and a perfect source of protein for those on a vegetarian diet.

Serves: 4
Preparation and cooking time:
approximately 25 minutes

340g/12oz fresh tofu
2 tbsp dark soy sauce
1 tbsp rice or sherry vinegar
1-2 tsp artificial sweetener
113g/4oz mangetout
1 large carrot
113g/4oz baby spinach
leaves
113g/4oz beansprouts
1 bunch spring onions
½ head Chinese leaves
2 tsp sesame oil
Chives to garnish

1. Drain and pat dry the tofu. Cut into small cubes and place in a bowl. Mix the soy sauce and vinegar together, and add sweetener to taste. Pour over the tofu, mix well and set aside while preparing the vegetables.

2. Top and tail the mangetout. Bring a small saucepan of water to the boil and cook the mangetout for 2 minutes until just tender but still slightly crisp. Drain and place under cold water to cool. Pat dry and place in another bowl.

3. Peel the carrot, and still using the peeler, shave pieces of carrot into the bowl. Wash and pat dry the spinach leaves and beansprouts and add to the bowl.

4. Trim the spring onions and halve lengthwise. Cut into shorter lengths and toss into the other vegetables.

5. To serve, shred the Chinese leaves and arrange on four serving plates. Drain the tofu, reserving the juices, and gently toss into the vegetables. Pile on top of the shredded leaves and spoon over the reserved juices. Finally drizzle each portion with a few drops of sesame oil and garnish with chives.

creamy potato and corn salad

Everyone loves potato salad, but usually it is served in a very fatty dressing. This version has a lighter dressing, but still retains the creaminess you'd expect from such a salad.

Serves: 4
Preparation time: approximately
10 minutes plus cooling
Cooking time: approximately
15 minutes

681g/1½lb baby or small salad potatoes
Salt and freshly ground black pepper
1 large leek
311g/11oz can sweetcorn kernels in water, drained and rinsed
4 tbsp very low-fat natural fromage frais
2 level tbsp low-calorie mayonnaise
2 tbsp freshly chopped dill

1. Place the potatoes in a large saucepan and cover with water. Add a pinch of salt and bring to the boil. Simmer for 10-12 minutes until tender. Drain well and allow to cool.

2. Meanwhile, trim the leek and slice in half lengthwise. Rinse under cold running water to flush out any trapped earth. Shred finely and place in a bowl. Mix in the sweetcorn, cover and chill until required.

3. Mix the remaining ingredients together, cover and chill until required.

4. Once the potatoes have cooled, mix into the leek and sweetcorn, and carefully mix in the dressing to serve.

grilled vegetable salad

If you think salad means two lettuce leaves and a slice of cucumber, read on. This heavy salad is full of chunky vegetables and makes a great lunch.

Serves: 4
Preparation and cooking time:
approximately 30 minutes

2 large baking potatoes,
each weighing around
283g/10oz
1 medium red pepper
1 medium yellow pepper
1 large red onion
1 large courgette
2 Little Gem lettuces

For the dressing:
6 tbsp lemon juice
1 garlic clove, peeled and
crushed
1 tsp dried mixed herbs
1-2 tsp granulated artificial
sweetener
Salt and freshly ground
black pepper

1. Scrub the potatoes and cut into slices approximately 1cm/½in thick. Bring to the boil in a large saucepan and cook for 6-7 minutes. Drain well.

2. Halve and de-seed the peppers and cut into thick wedges. Peel the onion and cut into thick wedges. Trim the courgette, slice lengthwise and cut into thick diagonal slices.

3. Preheat the grill on a high setting. Line a grill pan with foil and pile in the vegetables and potato slices – grill them in two batches if your grill pan is small.

4. Mix all the dressing ingredients together and sprinkle 2 tbsp over the vegetables. Grill for 7 minutes.

5. Turn the vegetables over and sprinkle over another 2 tbsp dressing. Grill for a further 7 minutes until lightly charred.

6. Discard any damaged outer leaves from the Little Gems, wash them and cut into quarters. Place on top of the vegetables. Sprinkle with remaining dressing and grill for 1-2 minutes until wilted and lightly browned.

7. Pile on to warmed serving plates and serve immediately.

Cook's Notes
This Syn-free dressing can also be tossed into cold salads.

You might prefer to use 1 tbsp fresh herbs in place of the dried.

layered sunshine salad

Here is a colourful and different way to serve a selection of salad vegetables. It is a particularly attractive dish to serve as part of a buffet.

Serves: 4
Preparation time: approximately
20 minutes plus chilling
Cooking time: approximately
10 minutes

4 medium eggs
113g/4oz radishes
1 small yellow or orange
pepper
1 small red onion
1 medium carrot
1 small head radicchio
lettuce or a few leaves of
other red lettuce such as
lollo rosso
1 tbsp lemon juice
2 tbsp fat-free vinaigrette
dressing
Freshly ground black pepper
¼ tsp paprika

1. Place the eggs in a small saucepan and cover with water. Bring to the boil and simmer gently for 8-10 minutes or until cooked to your liking - you do need the yolks to be quite firm for slicing. Drain and cool under cold running water. Set aside.

2. Wash and grate or finely slice the radishes. Halve and de-seed the pepper and cut into thin strips. Peel and finely slice or chop the red onion. Peel and grate the carrot or cut into thin strips. Discard any damaged outer leaves from the lettuce, wash and shake dry. Then cut into thin shreds.

3. Peel the eggs and cut into thin slices and place in the base of a 1.2 litre/2pt pudding basin, base lined with a circle of baking parchment. Now layer up the vegetables in any order you want, packing them down well, until the basin is full.

4. Mix the lemon juice and vinaigrette together and spoon over the top of the basin. Place a plate on top and weigh the top down with a 454g/1lb weight or a can of beans, etc. Place in the fridge for 1 hour.

5. To serve, remove the weight, invert the basin on to the plate and carefully lift the basin off. Season with black pepper and dust with paprika to serve.

middle eastern chickpea salad

The flavours in this filling and tasty salad are stronger because it is served cold. Serve it accompanied with boiled rice, bulgur wheat or couscous.

Serves: 4
Preparation and cooking time:
approximately 30 minutes
plus cooling

454g/1lb aubergines
1 large onion, peeled and finely chopped
1 garlic clove, peeled and crushed
142ml/¼pt vegetable stock
397g/14oz can chopped tomatoes
2 level tbsp tomato purée
1 tsp ground cinnamon
2 tsp granulated artificial sweetener
2 tbsp freshly chopped coriander
1 tbsp lemon juice
425g/15oz can chickpeas, drained and rinsed
Salt and freshly ground black pepper

1. Trim and dice the aubergines into 1cm/½in cubes. Place in a large saucepan and mix in the onion and garlic.

2. Pour in the stock and chopped tomatoes. Mix well. Bring to the boil and simmer gently, uncovered, for 20 minutes until softened. Set aside and allow to cool completely.

3. Stir in the remaining ingredients and season to taste. Transfer to a serving bowl, cover and chill for 1 hour before serving.

Cook's Notes

As a cheaper alternative you can use dried chickpeas. Soak 198g/7oz dried chickpeas overnight in a bowl of water, then rinse and simmer for 40-50 minutes or according to packet instructions.

salmon and asparagus salad

Salmon and asparagus complement one another perfectly. As you can prepare everything ready in advance, this dish makes an ideal quick lunch or supper.

Serves: 4

Preparation and cooking time: approximately 25 minutes plus cooling and chilling

4 x 170g/6oz salmon fillets
1 bay leaf
284ml/½pt vegetable stock
227g/8oz fine asparagus spears
Bunch of watercress
2 cartons of mustard and cress
¼ cucumber
Lemon wedges to garnish

For the dressing:
4 tbsp very low-fat natural fromage frais
5cm/2in piece cucumber, finely chopped
2 tbsp freshly chopped herbs such as parsley, tarragon and dill
½ tsp finely zested lemon rind
1 tbsp lemon juice
Salt and freshly ground black pepper

1. Using a sharp knife, cut the skin off the salmon. Wash and pat dry the fillets and place them in a frying pan with the bay leaf. Pour over the stock, bring to the boil, cover and simmer gently for 5-6 minutes until cooked through. Allow to cool, then drain and chill for 30 minutes.

2. Meanwhile, bring a large saucepan of water to the boil. Trim the woody ends from the asparagus, and then blanch the spears for 2-3 minutes until just tender. Drain and cool under cold running water. Chill until required.

3. Mix all of the dressing ingredients together and chill until required.

4. To serve, wash and trim the watercress and mustard and cress. Wash and thinly slice the cucumber. Line a large serving platter or four individual plates with these salads and then top with the chilled salmon and a few asparagus spears. Garnish with lemon wedges and serve with the herby dressing.

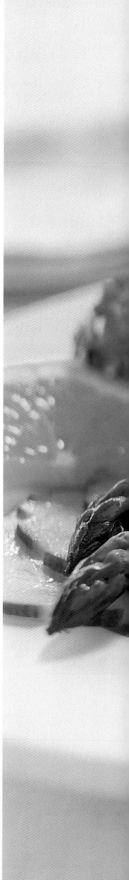

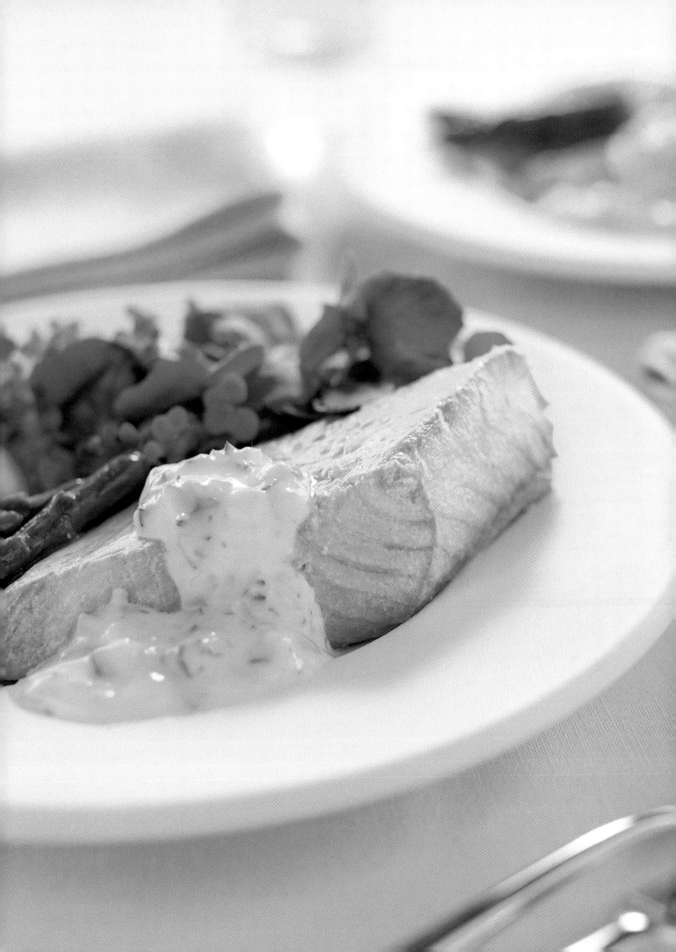

mixed bean salad

Beans are full of fibre and flavour, so make excellent, filling salad ingredients. Serve this salad with an egg dish or cold rice or pasta.

Serves: 4
Preparation time: approximately
10 minutes plus chilling
Cooking time: approximately
7 minutes

170g/6oz frozen green beans
113g/4oz frozen broad beans
Salt and freshly ground
black pepper
1 small red onion
425g/15oz can kidney beans
in water, drained and rinsed
397g/14oz can cannellini or
flageolet beans, drained and
rinsed
15g/½oz packet fresh basil
5 tbsp passata
1 tbsp red wine vinegar
1-2 tsp granulated artificial
sweetener

1. Bring a saucepan of lightly salted water to the boil and cook the frozen beans together for 5-6 minutes until tender. Drain well and rinse under cold water to cool, then pat dry and place in a large bowl.

2. Peel and finely slice the onion into thin rings. Mix into the cooked beans along with the canned beans. Season well.

3. Reserving a few small leaves for garnish, chop the remaining basil and mix into the beans.

4. Mix the passata and vinegar and add sufficient sweetener to taste. Toss into the beans. Cover and chill for 30 minutes before serving. Garnish with reserved basil leaves.

seafood niçoise salad

A substantial combination of assorted seafood, eggs and vegetables makes this a good main meal dish. You could serve it as a starter, in which case it would make six good portions.

Serves: 4

Preparation time: approximately 20 minutes

Cooking time: approximately 20 minutes

4 medium eggs
113g/4oz thin green beans
Salt and freshly ground black pepper
4 ripe medium plum tomatoes
1 cos lettuce
340g/12oz cooked mixed seafood, thawed if frozen
1 tbsp capers in brine, drained
28g/1oz pitted black olives in brine, drained
4 tbsp fat-free vinaigrette dressing
2 tbsp freshly chopped parsley

1. Place the eggs in a small saucepan and cover with water. Bring to the boil and simmer gently for 8-10 minutes or until cooked to your liking. Drain and cool in cold water.

2. Top and tail the green beans. Bring a small saucepan of lightly salted water to the boil and cook the beans for 6-7 minutes until just tender. Drain and cool in cold water.

3. Wash, dry and quarter the tomatoes. Discard any damaged outer leaves from the lettuce and rinse in cold water. Shake to remove excess water, then break into bite-sized pieces. Set aside.

4. In a bowl, mix together the seafood and capers. Slice the olives and mix into the seafood along with some seasoning.

5. Peel and quarter the eggs. Arrange the lettuce on four serving plates and top with green beans, tomatoes and eggs. Pile on the seafood and sprinkle with dressing and chopped parsley to serve.

turkey and cranberry salad

This Christmassy mixture of turkey and cranberry sauce is an excellent recipe to try at Christmas time when you're wondering how to use up the leftovers. Cooked chicken or ham would also make a good salad.

Serves: 4
Preparation time: approximately
20 minutes plus chilling

454g/1lb skinless lean cooked turkey meat
4 tbsp very low-fat natural fromage frais
2 level tbsp low-calorie mayonnaise
1 level tbsp cranberry sauce
Salt and freshly ground black pepper
1 bunch watercress
2 stalks celery with leaves
2 eating apples
1 tbsp lemon juice
1 large green pepper

1. Cut the turkey into bite-sized pieces and place in a bowl. Mix together the fromage frais, mayonnaise, cranberry sauce and seasoning and mix into the turkey. Cover and chill for 30 minutes.

2. Meanwhile, wash the watercress and shake to remove excess water. Trim and place in a large bowl. Reserving the celery leaves, trim and chop the stalks, and add to the watercress. Core and chop the apples. Toss in lemon juice. Halve, de-seed and chop the pepper and mix into the watercress along with the apples.

3. When ready to serve, pile the vegetables on to serving plates and top each portion with turkey mixture. Garnish with reserved celery leaves.

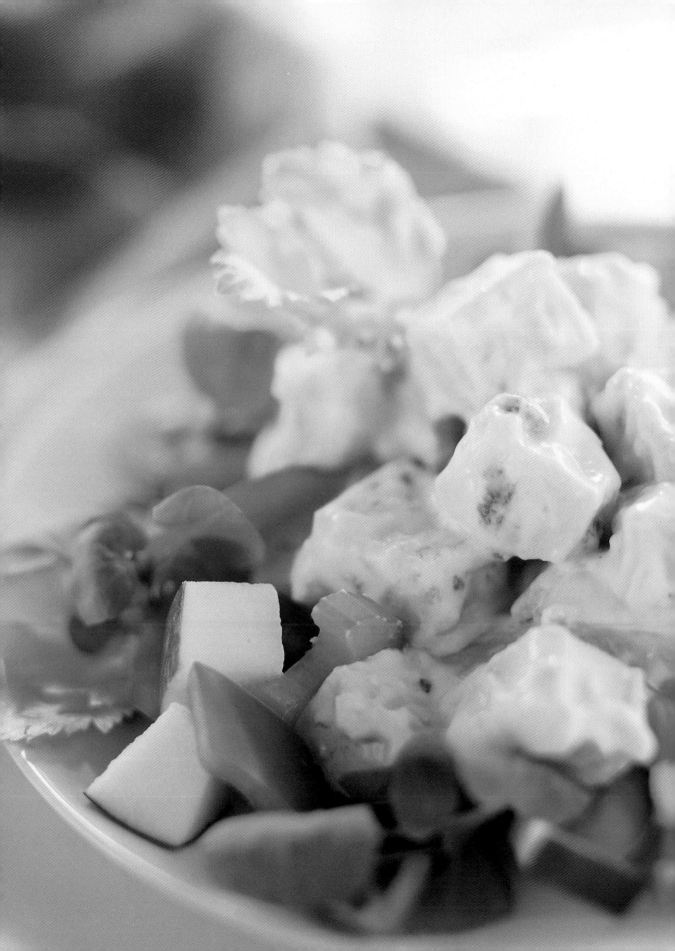

spicy cajun chicken salad

This salad is a quick snack meal or appetizer that is equally good made with hot or cold chicken. Served with a relish and a green salad it is a delicious combination of flavours.

Serves: 4
Preparation and cooking time:
approximately 25 minutes

2 tbsp American barbecue seasoning mix
1 tbsp ground paprika
1 tsp dried thyme
4 x 113g/4oz boneless skinned chicken breasts, washed
1 tsp vegetable oil
4 large beefsteak tomatoes, washed
1 small red onion
2 tbsp fresh chopped coriander
2 tsp red wine vinegar
1 tsp granulated artificial sweetener
Salt and freshly ground black pepper

1. Mix together the spices and dried thyme and place on a plate. Dip chicken on both sides lightly in the spices.

2. Brush a non-stick ridged frying pan with the oil and place on a high heat until very hot. Add the chicken, pressing down on the ridges to seal. Lower to a medium heat and cook the chicken for 7 minutes. Turn over and cook for a further 8 minutes or until cooked through.

3. Meanwhile, finely chop the tomato and place in a bowl. Peel and finely chop the onion and add to the tomato along with the remaining ingredients. Mix well and set aside.

4. Drain the chicken on absorbent kitchen paper, shred it into bite-sized pieces and serve with the relish, accompanied by a green salad.

sweet and sour pork salad

Here is an alternative way to serve this popular sweet and sour mix. The vegetables are not cooked, so they form a delicious, crunchy bed for the pork.

Serves: 4
Preparation and cooking time:
approximately 20 minutes

1 bunch spring onions
1 large red pepper
1 large carrot
½ medium fresh pineapple
170g/6oz beanshoots
454g/1lb lean pork fillet
1 garlic clove, peeled and
crushed
1 tsp Chinese five spice
powder
2 tsp vegetable oil
2 tbsp dark soy sauce
2 tbsp dry sherry

1. First prepare the vegetables. Trim and shred the spring onions. Halve, de-seed and dice the pepper. Peel and slice the carrot into thin matchstick pieces.

2. Slice the skin off the pineapple and remove the core if tough. Then dice the flesh. Mix all the vegetables together with the pineapple and beanshoots and pile on to four serving plates. Set aside.

3. Trim any excess fat and silver skin from the pork and then cut into thin shreds – the finer you slice the pork, the quicker it will cook.

4. Mix the pork with the garlic and five spice powder. Heat the oil in a non-stick wok until hot and stir-fry the seasoned pork for 4-5 minutes until cooked through. When piping hot, spoon pork over the prepared vegetables. Mix the soy sauce and sherry and pour over the pork and vegetables. Serve immediately.

warm herbed mushroom salad

With this really quick and easy recipe you can enjoy the subtle flavours of mushrooms cooked in herbs on crisp salad leaves.

Serves: 4
Preparation and cooking time:
approximately 15 minutes

681g/1½lb assorted firm mushrooms, such as large flat, chestnut, button, open cap and shiitake
1 garlic clove, peeled and crushed
1 bay leaf
1 tsp dried thyme
6 tbsp vegetable stock
Assorted salad leaves
4 tbsp freshly chopped parsley

For the dressing:
4 tbsp very low-fat natural fromage frais
1 tbsp red wine vinegar
1 tbsp granulated artificial sweetener
1 level tbsp wholegrain mustard
Salt and freshly ground black pepper

1. First prepare the mushrooms. Peel any mushrooms with a thick skin and wipe the others using absorbent kitchen paper. Cut the mushrooms so that they are more or less the same density: slice large flat mushrooms, quarter chestnut and open cap, halve shiitake, and keep button mushrooms whole, if very small.

2. Place the mushrooms in a large saucepan and add the garlic, bay leaf, thyme and stock. Cover, bring to the boil and cook over a medium to high heat, stirring occasionally, for 4-5 minutes until they are just cooked.

3. Meanwhile, line a salad bowl or serving plates with plenty of crisp salad leaves. Mix all the dressing ingredients together.

4. When the mushrooms are cooked, spoon over the leaves using a slotted spoon. Keep the mushroom stock for soups or stews. Spoon the dressing over the salads. Sprinkle chopped parsley over the whole salad. Serve immediately.

bolognese sauce

Here is a delicious low-fat version of everybody's favourite sauce to accompany pasta or spaghetti, depending on what you favour.

Serves: 4
Preparation and cooking time:
approximately 1 hour

1 onion
1 carrot
1 stick of celery
198g/7oz mushrooms
Fry Light
1 tsp chopped garlic
283g/10oz extra lean
minced beef
2 level tsp tomato purée
284ml/½ pint vegetable
stock
397g/14oz can chopped
tomatoes
Salt and freshly ground
black pepper, to taste

1. Prepare the vegetables: finely chop the onion, carrot and celery and roughly chop the mushrooms.

2. Heat a large non-stick saucepan and spray with Fry Light. Add the vegetables and garlic and cook for 5-6 minutes until the vegetables are soft, stirring often.

3. Add the minced beef and tomato purée and cook until the meat turns brown.

4. Add the stock, tomatoes and seasoning. Bring to the boil, reduce the heat and simmer gently for 45 minutes or until the meat is tender and the sauce is reduced. Check and adjust the seasoning and serve hot.

carbonara light

A traditional carbonara sauce is extremely high in fat but in our version we've reduced the fat levels drastically.

Serves: 4 as a starter
Preparation and cooking time:
approximately 20 minutes

1 small onion
1 clove garlic, crushed
2 tbsp vegetable stock
57g/2oz lean bacon
2 tbsp very low-fat natural
fromage frais
2 eggs
1 level tbsp grated
Parmesan cheese
2 tbsp chopped fresh flat
leaf parsley
Salt and pepper, to taste

1. Finely chop the onion and place in a non-stick saucepan with the garlic and stock. Gently cook for 4-5 minutes, stirring often. Remove all visible fat from the bacon, cut into thin strips, add to the pan and cook on high until the bacon is cooked through.

2. In a small bowl whisk together the fromage frais, eggs, Parmesan cheese, parsley and seasoning.

3. Cook the pasta of your choice, according to the packet instructions, drain and return to the pan on a very low heat. Add the bacon mixture and the egg mixture. Stir and cook for 2-3 minutes, spoon into warmed bowls and serve hot.

Cook's Note
The government advises that the elderly, babies and pregnant women should not eat raw eggs.

hot and spicy coleslaw

This is an ideal dish when preparing a low-fat feast when entertaining al fresco, or this dish makes a great jacket potato filling.

Serves: 4
Preparation time: approximately
20 minutes plus chilling

1 large carrot
113g/4oz each red and white cabbage
113g/4oz radishes
113g/4oz very low-fat natural yogurt
1 level tbsp horseradish sauce
3 tbsp freshly chopped chives
Salt and freshly ground black pepper

1. Peel and coarsely grate the carrot, finely shred the red and white cabbage and trim and thinly slice the radishes. Place all the vegetables into a bowl and mix.

2. Blend the yogurt, horseradish sauce, chives and seasoning, add to the bowl and mix.

3. Cover and chill for 30 minutes before serving to allow the flavours to develop.

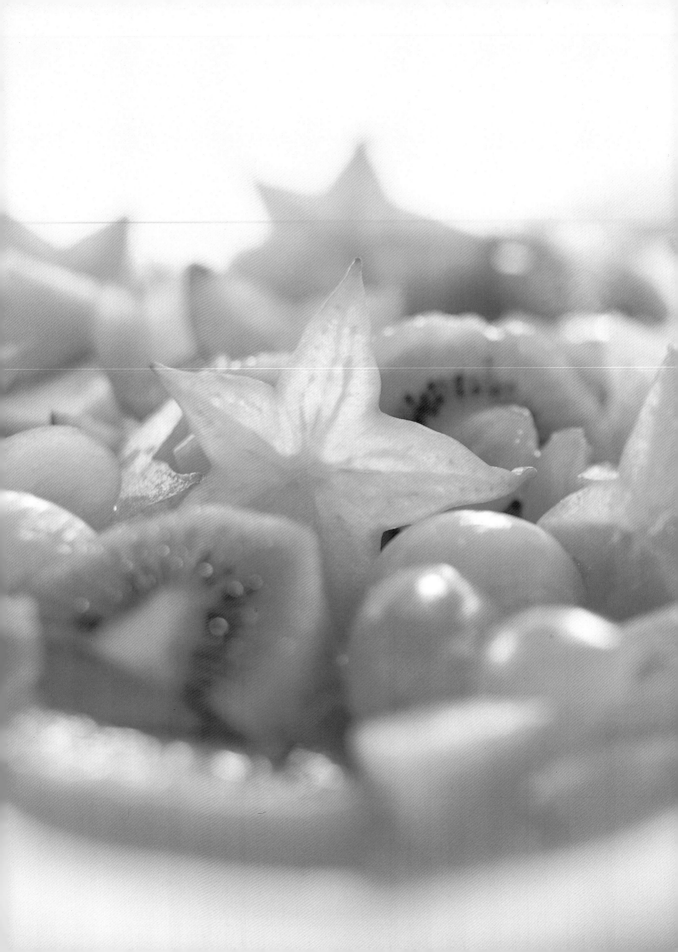

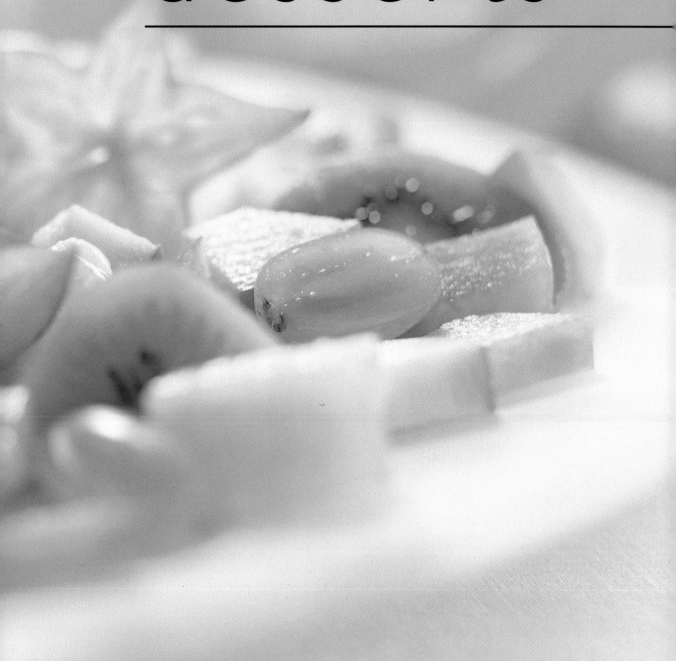

desserts

passion cake muffins

You can have your cake and eat it with these delicious low-fat muffins. They are topped with a sweetened quark frosting.

Makes: 8
Preparation and cooking time:
approximately 30 minutes plus
cooling time

3 medium eggs
6 tbsp granulated artificial sweetener
85g/3oz self-raising wholemeal flour
2 tsp ground mixed spice
170g/6oz grated carrot

Frosting:
113g/4oz quark skimmed milk soft cheese
1 tbsp granulated artificial sweetener
1 tsp vanilla essence

1. Preheat the oven to 180°/350°F/Gas 4. Line eight deep muffin tins with paper cases. In a large mixing bowl, whisk together the eggs and artificial sweetener until pale, thick and frothy – the mixture should be thick enough to hold a trail from the beaters.

2. Sieve in the flour and mixed spice, adding any husks that remain behind in the sieve. Add the carrot and, using a metal spoon, gently fold the ingredients together using a figure-of-eight action, taking care not to beat the mixture.

3. Spoon into the muffin cases to fill them and bake for 20 minutes until firm and lightly golden. Set aside to cool in the tin.

4. Meanwhile, make the frosting: beat together the three ingredients and chill in the fridge until required.

5. To serve, spread some of the frosting over each muffin and sprinkle with a little grated carrot to decorate.

Cook's Notes
Once frosted, store the muffins in the fridge. They will keep for 3-4 days – if you can leave them that long!

If preferred, replace the mixed spice with ground ginger or cinnamon for a different flavour.

minty apple cheesecake

This cheesecake has a ready-prepared base made from sponge fingers. The rich filling has a tangy flavour and light texture.

Serves: 6
Preparation time: approximately
20 minutes plus cooling and setting
Cooking time: approximately
10 minutes

454g/1lb cooking apples
Juice of 2 lemons
10 sponge fingers
1 sachet powdered gelatine
250g/9oz carton quark
skimmed milk soft cheese
255g/9oz very low-fat
natural fromage frais
2 tsp mint sauce
3-4 tbsp granulated artificial
sweetener
1 red-skinned eating apple
Mint leaves to decorate

1. Peel, core and chop the cooking apples. Place in a saucepan with half the lemon juice and 1 tbsp water. Bring to the boil, cover and simmer for 5 minutes until soft and pulpy. Allow to cool.

2. Meanwhile, line a 20cm/7in square tin with cling film so that it overlaps. Arrange the sponge fingers side by side in the bottom of the tin, trimming as necessary. Dissolve the gelatine in 4 tbsp boiling water and set aside to cool.

3. In a mixing bowl, beat together the quark, fromage frais and mint sauce. Add the cooled apple and add sweetener to taste. Stir in the gelatine and mix well. Spoon over the sponge fingers, smooth the top and chill for 2 hours until set.

4. Core the eating apple and cut into thin slices. Place in a small saucepan with the remaining lemon juice and gently bring to the boil. Cover and simmer for 2-3 minutes until just tender. Allow to cool.

5. To serve, carefully pull out the cheesecake from the tin and cut into six. Top each with a few slices of poached apple and mint leaves to decorate.

strawberry shortcake sundaes

This is just like having a slice of cheesecake in a glass! A simple yet very delicious and decadent dessert, it is also good made with raspberries.

Serves: 4
Preparation time: approximately
15 minutes

340g/12oz strawberries
283g/10oz very low-fat
natural fromage frais
A few drops almond essence
1-2 tbsp granulated artificial
sweetener
4 x butter crunch biscuits
4 x 57g/2oz scoops low-fat
vanilla ice cream

1. Reserving four strawberries for decoration, wash and hull the remaining, then slice thinly. Place half in a food processor or blender and blend for a few seconds until smooth.

2. Mix the fromage frais with sufficient almond essence and sweetener to taste.

3. Crush the biscuits finely.

4. To assemble, divide the sliced strawberries between four sundae glasses. Sprinkle over the crushed biscuits and then spoon in the fromage frais. Top with ice cream and a strawberry and serve immediately.

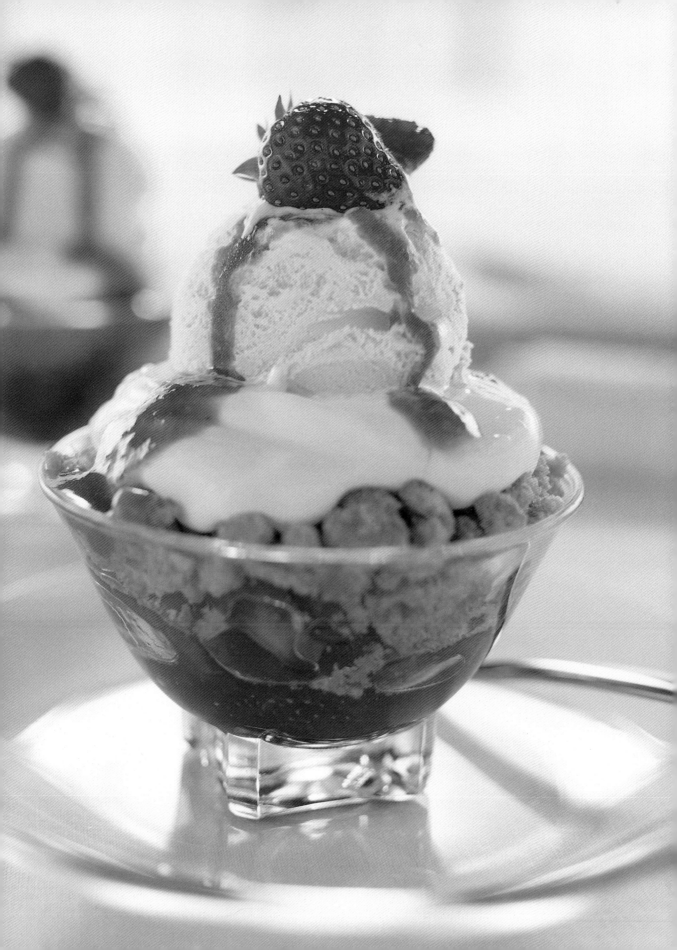

pineapple and mint cocktail

This sounds like an unusual combination, but it is very refreshing. Choose a pineapple that smells sweet through its skin, this denotes ripeness.

Serves: 4
Preparation time: 15 minutes plus
cooling and chilling

1 peppermint tea bag
1 large ripe pineapple
1-2 tsp granulated artificial sweetener
15g/¼oz packet fresh mint

1. Place the tea bag in a small heatproof jug and pour over 142ml/¼pt boiling water. Leave to infuse for 5 minutes, then remove the bag and allow the tea to cool.

2. Trim the leaves from the top of the pineapple and slice off the skin. Cut the flesh into bite-sized chunks, discarding the core if it is tough. Place in a bowl.

3. Add sufficient sweetener to the tea to taste and then pour over the fruit. Mix well, cover and chill for 30 minutes.

4. Just before serving, roughly chop the mint leaves. Pile the pineapple chunks on to serving plates or in glasses and sprinkle generously with mint. Accompany with fromage frais or yogurt to serve.

black forest ice cream

Although it takes time to make ice cream, this recipe is far nicer than anything you can buy in the shops, so it's well worth making the effort.

Serves: 4
Preparation time: approximately
15 minutes plus freezing and
standing

454g/1lb low-fat natural yogurt
3-4 tbsp granulated artificial sweetener
113g/4oz canned cherries, drained and rinsed
1 tbsp Kirsch
4 level tbsp double cream
142g/5oz very low-fat fromage frais
1 tsp vanilla essence
28g/1oz plain chocolate

1. Spoon the yogurt into a mixing bowl and stir in sweetener to taste.

2. Transfer the mixture to a large freezerproof container and place in the coldest part of your freezer. Allow to freeze for 1-1½ hours until the mixture is slushy. Beat well to break up the ice crystals.

3. Meanwhile, chop the cherries into small pieces. Mix in the Kirsch, then cover and chill until required.

4. Whip the cream until just peaking and fold into the fromage frais. Add the vanilla essence, cherries and Kirsch and then fold into the ice-cream mixture. Return to the freezer. Beat the mixture two to three times more at 30-40 minute intervals – this helps make a smoother, less icy ice cream. Then cover, seal and freeze until solid.

5. To serve, remove the ice cream 25-45 minutes before serving and allow to stand at room temperature until it becomes soft enough to spoon – this will depend on the temperature of your room. Scoop into serving dishes and grate the chocolate over to serve.

oriental green fruit salad

An attractive combination of subtle colours and flavours, this dish would make the perfect ending to a sophisticated dinner party.

Serves: 4
Preparation time: approximately
20 minutes plus cooling and chilling

1 Japanese green tea bag
1 lime
2 kiwi fruit
227g/8oz fresh lychees
¼ green-flesh melon such as
Gallia
113g/4oz seedless green
grapes
2 tbsp dry sherry
1-2 tsp granulated artificial
sweetener
Fresh lime to garnish

1. Place the tea bag in a small heatproof jug and pour over 142ml/¼pt boiling water. Leave to infuse for 5 minutes then discard the bag and allow the tea to cool, then cover and chill for 30 minutes.

2. Meanwhile, finely grate the rind from the lime and extract the juice. Set aside while preparing the fruit.

3. Peel and thinly slice the kiwi fruit. Peel, halve and stone the lychees. Remove the seeds from the melon and slice off the skin. Cut the flesh into small pieces. Wash and pat dry the grapes. Cover all the fruits and chill until required.

4. Once the tea has cooled, mix in the sherry, lime rind and juice and sufficient sweetener to taste.

5. To serve, arrange the fruits in small piles on four serving plates and drizzle over the tea mixture. Decorate with lime and serve.

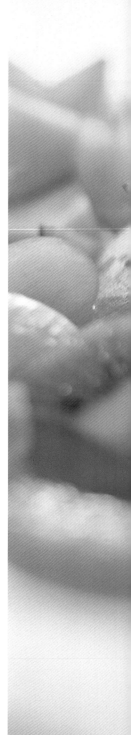

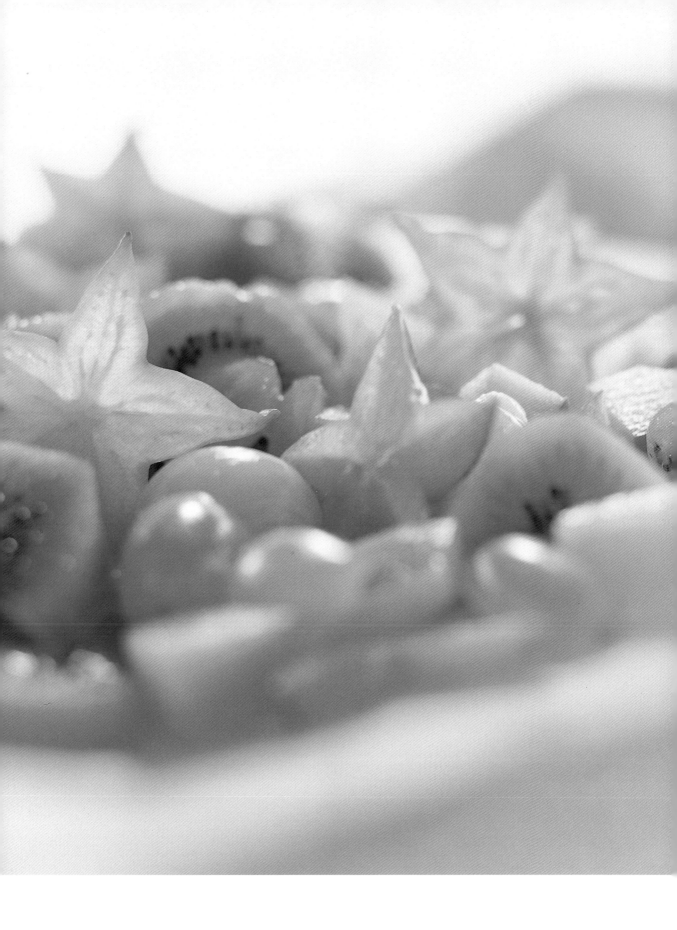

iced watermelon slices

This recipe would work just as well with other types of melon and try such flavourings as fresh grated root ginger or dried ground ginger instead of cinnamon. You may require less sweetener with other melons.

Serves: 4
Preparation and cooking time:
approximately 10 minutes
plus freezing

½ small watermelon,
weighing about 1.13kg/2½lb
Juice of 1 lemon
1 tsp ground cinnamon
3-4 tbsp granulated artificial
sweetener

1. Cut the watermelon lengthwise into four equal slices. Scoop out the flesh, reserving the shells, and place it in a blender or food processor with the lime juice. Process for a few seconds until smooth.

2. Place a sieve over a rigid freezerproof container and push the watermelon mixture through. Reserve a few seeds for decoration. Sweeten to taste: freeze for 2-2½ hours until slushy (this will depend on the depth of the watermelon in your container).

3. Meanwhile, place the reserved shells in a freezerproof bowl of matching size and reshape. Chill until required.

4. Beat the slushy watermelon mixture and refreeze for a further 2 hours. Turn into a chilled bowl and whisk until fluffy. Pile into the melon shell and smooth the top. Cover with foil and freeze until solid.

5. Place the watermelon bowl in a sink half-filled with hot water for 10 seconds or until the melon loosens. Carefully slide the melon out and stand on a plate at room temperature for 15-20 minutes until it begins to soften slightly.

6. Separate the melon wedges using a warmed knife and lay on a board lined with baking parchment. Pack the sorbet back into the slices if they have separated and push in a few of the reserved seeds to decorate. Replace in the freezer for 10 minutes to firm and then serve.

knickerbocker glories

They won't believe their eyes when they see these served up for pudding! The kids will love them – and they're low in fat too!

Serves: 4
Preparation time: approximately
15 minutes

2 kiwi fruit
170g/6oz raspberries,
thawed if frozen
2 x individual cartons ready
prepared strawberry-flavour
sugar-free jellies
198g/7oz carton very low-
fat natural fromage frais
1 tsp vanilla essence
1-2 tbsp granulated artificial
sweetener
8 x 28g/1oz scoops low-fat
chocolate ice cream
8 level tbsp low-fat aerosol
spray cream
2 level tsp chocolate flavour
ice-cream sauce
Mint sprigs to decorate

1. Peel the kiwi fruit and chop the flesh, then mix with all but four of the raspberries. Reserve the four for decoration.

2. Scoop out the jellies and mash lightly with a fork.

3. Mix the fromage frais with the vanilla and sufficient sweetener to taste.

4. To assemble, divide half the fruit between four tall serving glasses and top with a little jelly, fromage frais and a scoop of ice cream. Repeat the layers finishing with ice cream. Top each with a small squirt of cream and a drizzle of chocolate sauce. Decorate with mint and reserved raspberries. Serve immediately.

pimms cocktail jellies

A jelly for grown-ups! Bring back the flavours of summer with this fruity, set cocktail, and serve with a cucumber garnish for authenticity.

Serves: 4
Preparation time: approximately
20 minutes plus setting

1 sachet powdered gelatine
1 large orange
1 eating apple
Juice of 1 lemon
100ml/3½fl oz Pimms
426ml/¾pt diet lemonade
Lemon and cucumber slices
and mint sprigs to decorate

1. Pour 4 tbsp boiling water over the gelatine and stir until dissolved, then set aside.

2. Slice off the top and bottom from the orange, then slice off the skin taking away as much of the pith as possible. Slice in between each segment to release the flesh and place in a bowl with any juice that falls.

3. Core and finely chop the apple and toss in the lemon juice to prevent browning. Mix into the orange segments. Divide between four serving glasses.

4. Mix the Pimms with the gelatine and lemonade and pour over the fruit. Chill for 1-2 hours until set. Serve decorated with slices of lemon and cucumber, and sprigs of mint.

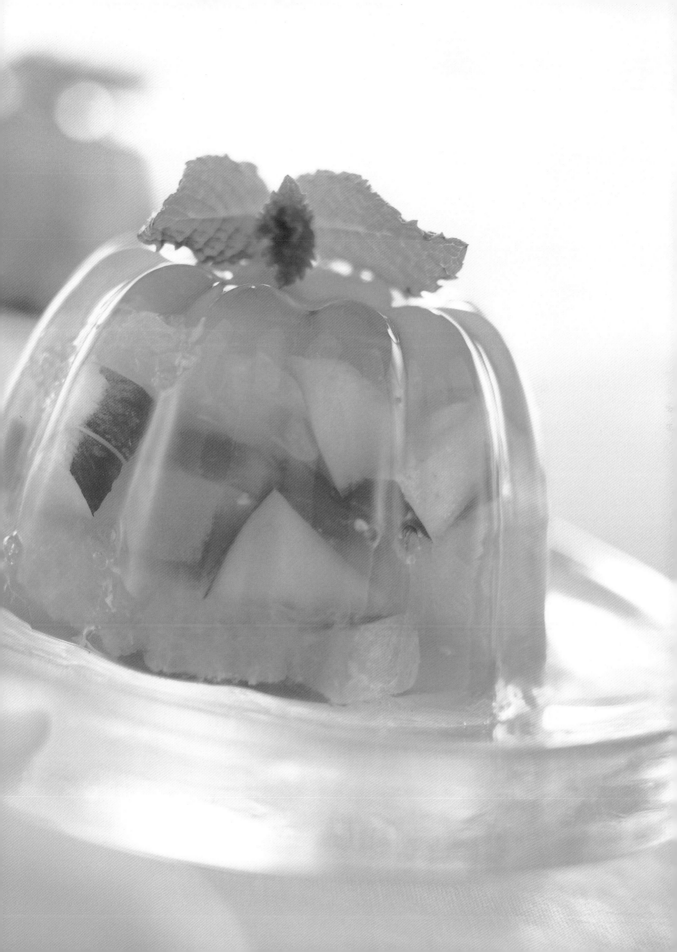

milk lollies

You can replace the milk with very low-fat natural yogurt if you prefer. This doesn't require thickening so you can omit the cornflour and the heating process.

Makes: 6

Preparation and cooking time: approximately 10 minutes plus freezing

568ml/1pt skimmed milk
3 tbsp granulated artificial sweetener
1 level tbsp cornflour

Suggested flavourings:
2 level tbsp low-calorie drinking chocolate
4 tbsp sugar-free fruit cordial
A few drops of peppermint essence
Food colouring (optional)

1. Mix 4 tbsp milk with the artificial sweetener and the cornflour. Pour the remaining milk into a saucepan and blend in the cornflour mixture. Heat, stirring, until boiling and slightly thickened. Remove from the heat and set aside to cool. If you are making the chocolate lollies, mix in the chocolate powder at this point. If using one of the other flavours, stir in to the cooled milk mixture and colour if desired.

2. Pour into six ice-lolly moulds (approximately 75ml/2½fl oz) and freeze until solid. Dip into hot water for a few seconds to unmould. Serve immediately.

speedy summer berry ice

Here is a super quick way to enjoy a homemade sorbet. Simply make sure you have everything at hand before you begin, and serve straight away.

Serves: 4
Preparation time: approximately
10 minutes

511g/1lb 2oz bag frozen
summer fruits
142ml/¼pt diluted Ribena,
no added sugar
113g/4oz very low-fat
natural fromage frais
2-3 tsp granulated artificial
sweetener
A few sprigs of mint
2 level tsp icing sugar

1. Just before you are ready to serve this dessert, place the fruits in a food processor or blender along with the diluted Ribena. Blend for a few seconds until well crushed and slightly slushy. You may have to blend the fruits a few times in order to crush them up.

2. Pile into serving glasses. Mix the fromage frais with sufficient sweetener and spoon over the berry ice. Decorate with mint and dust with icing sugar. Serve immediately.

Cook's Note
You can use you own assortment of fruit for this dessert, just make sure you choose small fruits like the berries and currants, and if you want to use larger soft fruits such as strawberries, cut them into smaller pieces before freezing, so that they will crush more easily.

lemon meringue pie

This delectable low-fat pud with a citrus kick is guaranteed to set your tastebuds tingling. The biscuit base and jelly crystal filling helps speed up the cooking time.

Serves: 6
Preparation and cooking time:
approximately 35 minutes
plus cooling and setting

12 Fox's Butter Crinkle Crunch Biscuits
3 egg whites
Juice and rind of 3 lemons
4 egg yolks
2 x 12g/½oz sachets sugar-free jelly crystals, lemon and lime
10 tbsp granulated artificial sweetener

1. Preheat the oven to 190°C/375°F/Gas 5. Line a 20.5cm/8in Victoria sandwich tin with baking parchment. Place the biscuits in a plastic bag and, holding the end closed, crush with a rolling pin.

2. In a bowl lightly beat one egg white, add the crushed biscuits and mix well. Transfer to the sandwich tin and press evenly over the base and up the sides using the back of a wetted spoon. Bake in the oven for 10 minutes, then set aside to cool.

3. Place the lemon juice and rind in a saucepan. Add 568ml/1pt water and whisk in the egg yolks. Heat, stirring continuously, until the mixture starts to thicken, taking care not to let it boil. Cook for a further 5 minutes. Remove from the heat and whisk in the jelly crystals and 4 tbsp artificial sweetener. Set aside to cool completely, then pour over the biscuit base. Chill for 2 hours until set, then carefully remove from the tin.

4. Whisk the remaining egg whites until they're very stiff and dry. Fold in the remaining artificial sweetener using a large metal spoon. Pile on top of the lemon filling, making sure that it is completely covered.

5. Place the lemon pie on a baking sheet and place under a preheated hot grill for about 1 minute until golden brown. Serve immediately.

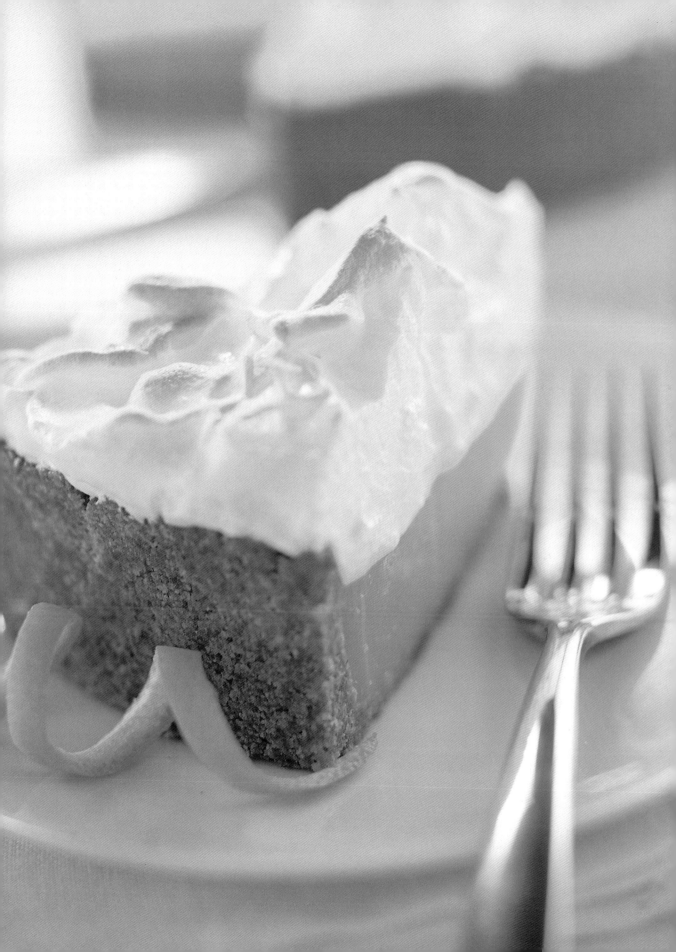

raspberry marshmallow meringues

Here is a particularly gooey, chewy dessert. The merginue base and raspberry topping complement one another perfectly.

Serves: 4
Preparation and cooking time:
approximately 30 minutes
plus cooling time

2 large egg whites
I level tsp cornflour
I tsp raspberry vinegar
113g/4oz light muscovado
sugar, free of lumps
142g/5oz very low-fat
natural fromage frais
227g/8oz raspberries,
thawed if frozen
Artificial sweetener, to taste

1. Preheat the oven to 160°C/325°F/Gas 2. In a large grease-free bowl, whisk the egg white until very stiff and dry. Add the cornflour and vinegar and gradually whisk in the sugar, a spoonful at a time, until the mixture is stiff again.

2. Line a large baking sheet with baking parchment and divide the mixture into four even mounds on the tray. Smooth each into a round with a diameter of approximately 10cm/4in. Then bake in the oven for 20 minutes until firm on the outside. Allow to cool – the marshmallows will shrink down on cooling.

3. To serve, remove each marshmallow from the paper using a pallet knife and arrange on serving plates. Top with fromage frais and a few raspberries. Place the remaining raspberries in a sieve over a bowl and press through to extract the juice. Sweeten to taste and spoon over the marshmallows to serve.

blackberry and apple tansy

A traditionally West Country pudding made from eggs, this is really a sweet omelette with fruit set in it. It's very light and has a melt-in-the-mouth texture.

Serves: 4

Preparation time: approximately 10 minutes

Cooking time: approximately 15 minutes

454g/1lb cooking apples
Juice of 1 lemon
227g/8oz blackberries,
thawed of frozen
4 medium eggs
1 tsp ground cinnamon
4 tbsp skimmed milk
2-3 tbsp granulated artificial
sweetener
1 level tbsp icing sugar

1. Peel, core and cut the apples into thin wedges. Place in a small saucepan and toss in the lemon juice and 1 tbsp water. Bring to the boil, cover and simmer for 3-4 minutes until just tender but still holding their shape.

2. Transfer the apples to a medium-sized non-stick frying pan using a draining spoon and arrange evenly over the bottom of the pan. Sprinkle over the blackberries.

3. Beat the eggs together with the cinnamon, milk and sweetener to taste. Pour over the fruit. Cook over a medium heat for 7-8 minutes until just set.

4. Preheat the grill to a hot setting. Thickly dust the egg with icing sugar and place under the grill to cook for 1-2 minutes until lightly golden and caramelized.

5. Serve hot, cut into wedges, accompanied with fromage frais.

Cook's Note
If blackberries are unavailable, raspberries would make an excellent and colourful alternative.

cappuccino pots

Impress you guests and serve these light coffee mousses in small coffee cups for maximum effect. The government advises that the elderly, babies and pregnant women should not eat raw eggs.

Serves: 4
Preparation time: approximately 15 minutes plus setting

2 tsp powdered gelatine
5 level tbsp low-fat crème fraîche
9 tbsp very low-fat natural fromage frais
1 tbsp coffee and chicory essence
3 tbsp granulated artificial sweetener
2 large egg whites
4 chocolate coffee beans
1 level tsp drinking chocolate

1. Pour 2 tbsp boiling water over the gelatine and stir until dissolved, then set aside.

2. Place the crème fraîche together with 5 tbsp fromage frais in a bowl and mix in the coffee essence and sweetener. In another bowl, whisk the egg white until stiff.

3. Mix the gelatine into the coffee mixture and fold in the egg whites. Divide the mixture between four cups or serving glasses. Chill for 1-2 minutes until set.

4. To serve, spoon the remaining fromage frais on top, decorate each with a coffee bean and sprinkle lightly with drinking chocolate.

chocolate egg custards

These chocolate egg custards are a traditional dessert with a touch of decadence by the addition of chocolate. Serve simply with fresh fruit.

Serves: 4
Preparation time: approximately
10 minutes
Cooking time: approximately
25 minutes

340g/12oz very low-fat
natural fromage frais
28g/1oz cocoa powder
1 tsp vanilla essence
1-2 tbsp granulated artificial
sweetener
3 large eggs

1. Preheat the oven to 180°C/350°F/Gas 4. Place the fromage frais in a bowl and sieve in the cocoa powder. Stir in the vanilla and sufficient sweetener to taste.

2. Beat the eggs together and mix into the chocolate fromage frais.

3. Place four ovenproof ramekin dishes in a roasting tin. Divide the egg mixture between the dishes and pour sufficient boiling water into the roasting tin to come half way up the sides of the dishes.

4. Bake in the oven for 25 minutes until set. Serve hot or cold with strawberries or other fruits.

Cook's Note
If you cool and chill the custards, they will be firm enough to turn out before serving.

chocolate orange mousse

This easy-to-prepare mousse uses ready-prepared orange jelly crystals; it is the perfect partner for chocolate, and is sure to be popular.

Serves: 4
Preparation time: approximately
20 minutes plus cooling and chilling

1 x 14.5g/½oz sachet sugar-free orange jelly crystals
500g/1lb 2oz carton very low-fat natural fromage frais
28g/1oz cocoa powder
2 large egg whites
1-2 tbsp granulated artificial sweetener
2 large oranges
28g/1oz plain chocolate

1. Dissolve the jelly crystals in 142ml/¼pt boiling water and set aside to cool completely.

2. Place the fromage frais in a bowl and sieve in the cocoa powder. In another bowl whisk the egg whites until stiff.

3. Whisk the cooled jelly into the fromage frais and add sufficient sweetener to taste. Fold in the egg whites and either spoon into four serving dishes or one large dish. Chill for 1-2 hours until set.

4. Meanwhile, slice the top and bottom off each orange and slice off the peel, taking away as much of the white pith as possible. Slice in between each segment to release the flesh. Cover and chill until required.

5. To serve, arrange a few slices of orange on top of each mousse and grate over the chocolate.

Cook's Note
The government advises that the elderly, babies and pregnant women should not eat raw eggs.

pashka

Here is a dessert based on a rich cream cheese and butter Russian dessert traditionally served at Easter time. This lighter version is excellent served with fresh fruit when you want something a bit more special than fromage frais.

Serves: 4
Preparation time: approximately
15 minutes plus draining

255g/9oz very low-fat natural cottage cheese
255g/9oz very low-fat natural fromage frais
1 tsp vanilla essence
3 tbsp granulated artificial sweetener
2 medium egg whites
57g/2oz luxury dried fruit mix
1 tsp finely grated lemon rind

1. Place a sieve over a bowl and push the cottage cheese through using the back of a spoon. Mix in the fromage frais, vanilla essence and sweetener.

2. Whisk the egg whites until stiff and fold into the cheese mixture along with the dried fruit and lemon rind.

3. Pile the mixture into the centre of a large piece of clean, white muslin or a clean, plain tea towel. Bring up the sides and twist the top together tightly to lightly squeeze the cheese inside and secure with string. Place on top of a large jug or small bowl to catch the liquid that will drip and chill for 2-4 hours until drained and firm.

4. Scrape the cheese into a bowl and then scoop on to serving plates. Serve accompanied with assorted fresh fruits.

tropical fruit rice pudding

Liven up rice pudding with a touch of coconut and some fresh fruit. This super speedy rice pudding is made on top of the oven rather than baked, so you can make it in next to no time.

Serves: 6
Preparation time: approximately
15 minutes plus cooling
Cooking time: approximately
20 minutes

170g/6oz shortgrain rice
14g/½oz block creamed coconut
198g/7oz very low-fat natural fromage frais
1 tsp vanilla essence
2-3 tbsp granulated artificial sweetener
1 small ripe mango
1 large banana
1 lime
1 small pineapple

1. Place the rice in a sieve and rinse under cold water until the water runs clear. Place in a saucepan and pour over 568ml/1pt water. Grate the coconut into the saucepan. Bring to the boil, then simmer gently, uncovered, for 15-20 minutes until the rice is soft and the water is absorbed. Stir the mixture occasionally and keep the heat low to prevent sticking.

2. Remove from the heat and transfer to a heatproof bowl. Stir in the fromage frais, vanilla essence and add sweetener to taste. Allow to cool.

3. Meanwhile, peel the mango and slice down either side of the smooth, flat, central stone. Discard the stone and chop the flesh and place in a bowl. Peel and slice the banana and mix into the mango. Finely grate the lime rind into the fruit and extract the juice, and toss in. Finally, peel, slice and chop the pineapple and mix into the other fruits. Cover and chill until required.

4. Serve the rice pudding with the tropical fruit salad, with extra lime to squeeze over if liked.

Cook's Note
If preferred, you can serve the rice as soon as it is cooked for a delicious hot pudding.

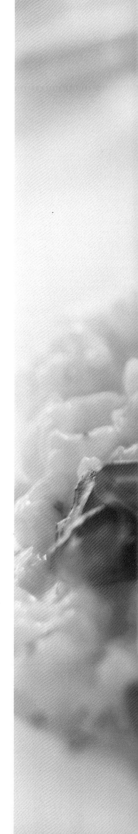

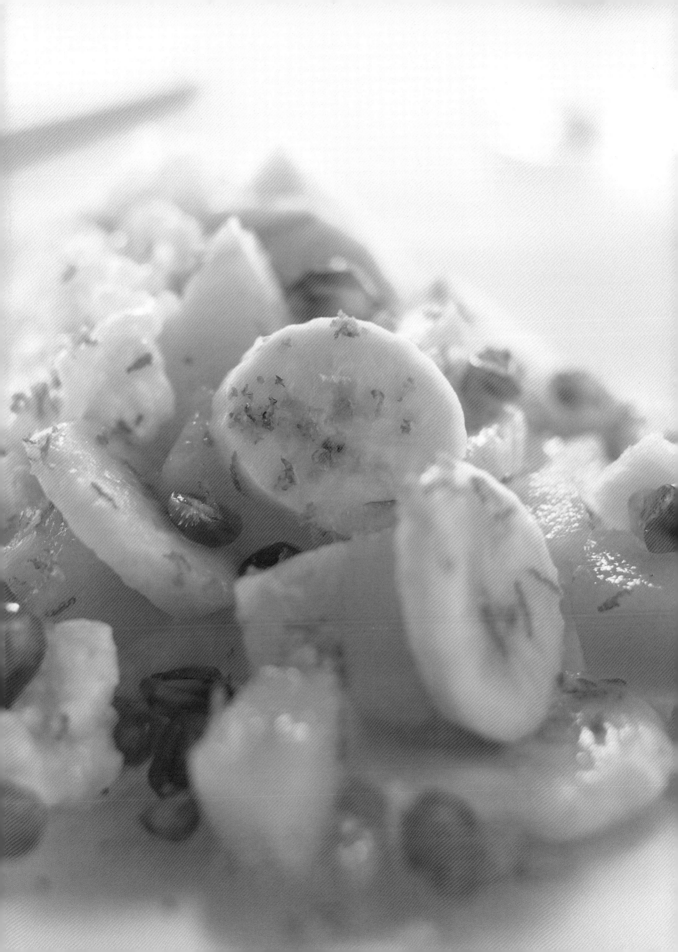

tiramisu

Think the tiramisu is off the menu when losing weight? Think again! With a few simple low-fat switches, our slimline version of this classic Italian dessert looks and tastes sensational.

Serves 6
Preparation and cooking time:
approximately 20 minutes
plus chilling

2 medium egg yolks
3 tbsp granulated artificial sweetener
Few drops vanilla essence to taste
397g/14oz quark skimmed milk soft cheese
12 sponge fingers
2 tsp instant coffee dissolved in 2 tbsp water
2 tbsp brandy
142g/5oz very low-fat natural fromage frais
12 chocolate-covered coffee beans
2 level tsp cocoa powder

1. In a mixing bowl, whisk together the egg yolks and 2 tbsp sweetener until thick and creamy. Add the vanilla essence and 2 tbsp quark and whisk in gently. Gradually whisk in the remaining quark to form a smooth cream.

2. Break the sponge fingers in half and place them in a shallow dish. Mix the coffee and brandy together and drizzle over the sponge fingers, mixing them gently to coat in the liquid.

3. Divide half of the sponge fingers between six small serving glasses, top with half the cream mixture, then with the rest of the sponge fingers and a second layer of cream. Chill for 30 minutes.

4. To serve, sweeten the fromage frais with the remaining sweetener and spoon on top of each glass. Decorate with coffee beans and dust with cocoa.

apple and apricot bake

This satisfying pudding combines fresh fruit with canned, and will certainly be popular with all the family. It only takes 8 minutes to cook so it can be baking while you eat your main course.

Serves: 4
Preparation time: approximately
15 minutes
Cooking time: approximately
8 minutes

454g/1lb cooking apples
Juice of 1 lemon
397g/14oz can apricot halves
in natural juice, drained
3-4 tbsp granulated artificial
sweetener
4 slices wholemeal Nimble
bread
14g/½oz low-fat spread
½ tsp ground cinnamon

1. Peel, core and chop the apples and place them in a saucepan. Toss the lemon juice into the apples along with 1 tbsp water. Gently bring to the boil, cover and simmer for 5 minutes until soft and pulpy.

2. Meanwhile, slice the apricots and stir into the apple along with sufficient sweetener to taste. Set aside.

3. Preheat the grill to a hot setting and toast the bread lightly on each side until golden brown.

4. Spread the toasted bread on one side with a light covering of low-fat spread and then sprinkle with cinnamon and sweetener. Return to the grill and cook for a few seconds further until bubbling and richly golden.

5. To serve, reheat the fruit if necessary. Cut the bread into small triangles and serve a portion of fruit with the toasted spiced bread on top.

chunky bread pudding

A real school-days pudding. This hearty dish of bread soaked in a thick, set custard has a hint of spice and fruitiness. It's a real treat.

Serves: 6
Preparation time: approximately
10 minutes plus standing
Cooking time: approximately
40 minutes

4 x 57g/2oz soft wholemeal
bread rolls
57g/2oz sultanas
6 medium eggs
500g/1lb 2oz very low-fat
natural fromage frais
1 tsp ground mixed spice
2-3 tbsp granulated artificial
sweetener

1. Preheat the oven to 180°C/350°F/Gas 4. Cut the bread rolls into small cubes and place in an ovenproof shallow gratin dish. Sprinkle over the sultanas.

2. Beat the eggs together and mix into the fromage frais. Add the spice and sufficient sweetener to taste.

3. Spoon the fromage frais custard over the bread and turn the bread over in the custard to make sure it is completely covered.

4. Stand the dish in a roasting tin and pour sufficient boiling water into the tin to come halfway up the sides of the gratin dish. Bake in the oven for 35-40 minutes until set and a knife inserted in the centre comes out clean.

5. Remove the dish from the tin and stand for 10 minutes before serving, sprinkled with extra sweetener if liked.

pear and raspberry crisp

This crunchy topping livens up lightly cooked fruit to make a colourful and very delicious pudding. It is also good made with blackberries and apple.

Serves: 4
Preparation time: approximately
15 minutes
Cooking time: approximately
12 minutes

4 ripe pears
1 lemon
227g/8oz raspberries,
thawed if frozen
2-3 tsp granulated artificial
sweetener
42g/1½oz cornflakes
4 level tsp maple syrup
28g/1oz low-fat spread

1. Core and peel the pears. Cut into thick wedges and place in a large saucepan. Finely grate the lemon zest into the saucepan and add the lemon juice. Mix the pears in the juice until well coated.

2. Pour in 142ml/¼pt water. Bring to the boil, cover and simmer for 5 minutes. Add the raspberries and mix gently together. Continue to cook, covered, for a further 2-3 minutes until tender. Add sweetener to taste then transfer the fruit to an ovenproof dish.

3. Place the cornflakes in a mixing bowl. Place the maple syrup and low-fat spread in a small saucepan and melt over a very low heat. Toss into the cornflakes and stir until well coated. Scatter on top of the fruit to lightly cover it.

4. Preheat the grill to a hot setting and cook the fruit crisp for 1-2 minutes until the topping is bubbling and lightly golden.

strawberry and raspberry filo slices

This is an impressive-looking dessert which needs eating quickly to enjoy it at its best. So assemble it at the last minute before serving.

Serves: 4
Preparation time: approximately
20 minutes plus cooling
Cooking time: approximately
10 minutes

3 x 28g/1oz large sheets
frozen filo pastry, thawed
1 medium egg, beaten
113g/4oz small strawberries
113g/4oz raspberries,
thawed if frozen
283g/10oz very low-fat
natural fromage frais
1 tsp almond essence
1-2 tbsp granulated artificial
sweetener
2 level tsp icing sugar
Mint to decorate

1. Preheat the oven to 200°C/400°F/Gas 6. Lay the sheets of filo on the work surface and brush with beaten egg. Fold over lengthwise, brush with more egg and fold again. You should have three long strips.

2. Cut the strips into four equal portions and lay side by side on a baking sheet lined with baking parchment. Brush with more egg and bake for 8-10 minutes until golden brown. Carefully remove from the paper and allow to cool on a wire rack.

3. Meanwhile, wash, hull and halve the strawberries. Mix with the raspberries, cover and chill. Mix the fromage frais with almond essence and sufficient sweetener to taste. Cover and chill until required.

4. To serve, place a piece of crisp pastry on each of four serving plates. Spread with half the fromage frais and fruit. Lay another sheet on top and repeat with remaining fromage frais and fruit. Finally place the remaining pastry on top, dust with icing sugar and decorate with mint to serve. Serve immediately.

Cook's Note
These pastries are best served as soon as they are assembled, otherwise the pastry may soften.

tropical fruit baskets

These crisp filo pastry cases are filled with a creamy coconut fromage frais mixture. Fill the cases just before serving to prevent them softening.

Serves: 4

Preparation time: approximately 20 minutes plus cooling

Cooking time: approximately 10 minutes

2 x 28g/1oz large sheets frozen filo pastry, thawed
1 medium egg, beaten
1 small ripe papaya
1 small pineapple
1 small ripe mango
1 tbsp dark rum
1 level tbsp dark brown sugar
227g/8oz very low-fat natural fromage frais
14g/½oz block creamed coconut
1-2 tsp granulated artificial sweetener

1. Preheat the oven to 200°C/400°F/Gas 6. Lay the sheets of pastry on top of each other and cut into six equal pieces. Gently press one piece of pastry into the base of four deep muffin tins. Brush with a little egg and press another piece on top at a different angle. Brush again and top with the remaining pastry. Push in the edges slightly to create a case.

2. Brush with more egg and bake in the oven for 8-10 minutes until crisp and golden. Cool for 10 minutes, then remove from the tin and place on a wire rack to cool completely.

3. Meanwhile, prepare the filling. Peel the papaya. Cut in half and scoop out the seeds. Chop the flesh into small pieces and place in a bowl. Peel, slice and cube the pineapple. Peel the mango and slice down either side of the smooth, flat, central stone. Discard the stone and chop the flesh. Mix into the papaya along with the pineapple and rum. Cover and chill until required.

4. Mix the brown sugar with the fromage frais. Finely grate the coconut into the fromage frais and add sweetener if necessary. Cover and chill until required.

5. To serve, place the pastry cases on serving plates and fill with fromage frais. Top with some of the fruit, and serve the remaining as an accompaniment.

griddled maple lemon pears

Griddles are really useful for low-fat cooking, though they aren't normally used for cooking fruit!
Give it a try – we think the result tastes and looks gorgeous!

Serves: 4
Preparation and cooking time:
approximately 20 minutes

1 large lemon
4 ripe dessert pears
2 level tbsp maple syrup
170g/6oz very low-fat
natural fromage frais
1 tbsp granulated artificial
sweetener
Mint to decorate

1. Finely grate the rind and extract the juice from the lemon. Reserve the rind, place the juice in a large bowl.

2. Peel the pears, cut in half through the stalk and toss in the lemon juice – this will help prevent browning.

3. Heat a non-stick ridged or flat griddle pan until hot. Press the pear halves, four at a time, on to the pan, and drizzle each with a little of the maple syrup. Cook for 20-30 seconds to seal, turn over and repeat. Transfer to a warmed serving dish and keep warm. Repeat with remaining pear slices and maple syrup.

4. Mix the fromage frais with sweetener and sufficient lemon rind to taste. Serve warm pear slices with the lemon fromage frais, sprinkled with any remaining lemon rind. Decorate with mint and serve immediately.

Cook's Note
The pears must be ripe for the recipe otherwise they will require longer cooking, and this would mean that the maple syrup would burn. To check if the pears are ripe, they should feel slightly soft when squeezed. They will also yield juice once cut.

ginger banoffee pudding

Banoffee pudding – made with bananas and toffee yogurt – is an old favourite with Slimming World members. We've given it a twist with ginger biscuits – and best of all, it's ready in 10 minutes. Prepare it just before serving so that the banana stays fresh.

Serves: 4
Preparation time: approximately 10 minutes

6 ginger nut biscuits
2 large bananas
1 tbsp lemon juice
4 x 200g/7oz tubs Müllerlight toffee yogurt
14g/½oz plain chocolate, grated

1. Place the ginger biscuits in a clean plastic bag. Seal and crush finely with a rolling pin.

2. Peel and thinly slice the bananas, then toss in the lemon juice to prevent browning.

3. Layer the toffee yogurt, sliced banana and crushed ginger biscuits alternating in four serving glasses. Top each glass with a sprinkling of grated chocolate and serve.

recipe syn values

The Syns given for each of the recipes in this book are per portion for both Original and Green days, unless otherwise specified.

STARTERS	Page no.	Original Day	Green Day
Chicken gumbo	59	1½	10
Chicken tikka	78	Free	7½
Chinese chicken and mushroom soup	62	1	8½
Classic leek and potato soup	63	6	Free
Crispy potato skins	79	2	Free
French-style fish soup	66	1½	13½
Gazpacho with prawns	67	Free	4½
Gingered vegetable filo parcels	58	3½	3½
Hearty bean and vegetable soup	68	11	Free
Insalata di mare	74	Free	9
Italian-style bacon soup with pesto	64	1	3
Mexican avocado dip	54	2	2
Middle Eastern spiced lentil broth	69	4	Free
Mixed root vegetable soup	70	2½	½
Mushrooms à la greque	56	1	1
Peperonata filo tarts	60	3	3
Prawn and melon cocktail	72	1	9½
Roast Mediterranean vegetable soup	71	Free	Free
Smoked fish pâté	75	2	14½
Spinach roulade with red pepper sauce	55	serves 4: 1 serves 6: ½	serves 4: 1 serves 6: ½
Terrine of chicken	76	1	11
Waldorf stuffed pear with Parma ham	77	2	8

MAIN COURSES: MEAT	Page no.	Original Day	Green Day
Caribbean pork	99	3	11½
Chicken and pumpkin casserole	86	1	10
Chicken Kiev	87	2½	10
Chicken korma	88	3	12
Chicken with peaches and raspberries	89	5½	13
Corned beef hash	106	1½	8
Garlic chicken and vegetable pot roast	90	Free	10½
Hot chicken sandwich	94	Free	7½
Kleftico-style lamb steaks	96	Free	11½
Lemon chicken with artichokes	91	2	9½

Mango duck with mustard mash	95	I	I6
Meatloaf with spinach and pepper stuffing	82	I	I6
Mustard pork steaks with red cabbage and apple	I02	2	9
Pizzaiola steak	83	I	I3
Pork and herb meatballs with ratatouille sauce	I04	Free	7
Redcurrant lamb with leek and swede mash	I00	2½	I0½
Roast lamb with a curried crust	98	½	I6
Steak and mushroom pie	I07	4	I6
Teriyaki beef and orange skewers	84	2½	I0½
Thai green chicken curry	92	3	9
Turkey satay with peanut sauce	I03	4	I0

MAIN COURSES: FISH	**Page no.**	**Original Day**	**Green Day**
Cajun griddled fish	II0	Free	9
Cod in parsley sauce	III	I	8½
Greek fish wrapped in vine leaves	II4	½	monkfish: 6½
			cod: 8
			halibut: 9½
Monkfish and bacon kebabs	II5	Free	6
Pan-cooked prawns with garlic and vermouth	II2	I½	4½
Plaice and salmon rolls	II6	I	9½
Ribbon trout	II8	Free	9½
Salmon Florentine	II9	I	I3½

MAIN COURSES: VEGETARIAN	**Page no.**	**Original Day**	**Green Day**
Baked couscous pudding with chunky chilli vegetable sauce	I31	II	Free
Beany sausages and tomato sauce	I43	5½	Free
Cassoulet	I40	I2½	I½
Chilli Quorn, sweetcorn and pepper kebabs	I32	5½	Free
Curried lentil and Quorn burgers	I29	5½	Free
Indian-style rice and split peas	I34	I4½	½
Macaroni cheese stuffed peppers	I22	8½	I
Mexican green rice	I35	I7	Free
Mushroom cannelloni	I23	I9	2½
Mushroom stroganoff	I4I	½	½
Noodles with shredded ginger vegetables	I26	II½	I½
Pasta timbales	I24	9	I½
Pasta with special pesto	I27	I6	I
Pastitso	I30	8	I
Pumpkin risotto	I38	I7	2
Quorn chilli with spicy potato wedges	I47	I4	Free
Ratatouille with eggs	I44	Free	Free

Root vegetable and lentil casserole	142	8	Free
Spanish-style tortilla	145	6	Free
Spicy tabbouleh with apricots	139	19½	3
Sweetcorn pasta bake	146	17	3
Vegetable lasagne	128	8	4½

VEGETABLES AND SALADS	**Page no.**	**Original Day**	**Green Day**
Artichoke and cherry tomato salad	166	1½	1½
Bolognese sauce	181	½	6½
Carbonara light	182	½	1½
Cauliflower and potato curry	155	5½	1½
Chinese vegetable salad	167	1	1
Creamy potato and corn salad	168	12½	1½
Dolmades	158	½	Free
Fruity coronation chicken	150	2½	12½
Garlic and rosemary roast baby potatoes	159	8	Free
Grilled vegetable salad	169	5	Free
Ham and pineapple rolls	151	Free	7½
Hot and spicy coleslaw	183	½	½
Layered sunshine salad	170	Free	Free
Maple baked roots	162	6½	2½
Middle Eastern chickpea salad	171	6	½
Mini-lamb koftas	154	Free	2
Mixed bean salad	174	10½	Free
Mustard baked potato wedges	163	1½	½
Roast beef with Mexican-style coleslaw	152	Free	7½
Salmon and asparagus salad	172	Free	15
Seafood niçoise salad	175	½	4
Slimming World's syn-Free chips	156	8	Free
Spicy Cajun chicken salad	178	½	6½
Spicy red roast vegetables	160	½	½
Stir-fried summer vegetables	164	½	½
Sweet and sour pork salad	179	1½	8½
Turkey and cranberry salad	176	1½	10½
Warm herbed mushroom salad	180	½	½

DESSERTS	**Page no.**	**Original Day**	**Green Day**
Apple and apricot bake	211	7	7
Black forest ice cream	191	7	7
Blackberry and apple tansy	203	3½	3½
Cappuccino pots	204	3	3
Chocolate egg custards	205	1	1
Chocolate orange mousse	206	3½	3½

Chunky bread pudding	212	5½	5½
Ginger banoffee pudding	217	4½	4½
Griddled maple lemon pears	216	4½	4½
Iced watermelon slices	194	2½	2½
Knickerbocker glories	195	5	5
Lemon meringue pie	200	5½	5½
Milk lollies	198	2	2
with drinking chocolate:		3	3
Minty apple cheesecake	187	3½	3½
Oriental green fruit salad	192	½	½
Pashka	207	2	2
Passion cake muffins	186	1½	1½
Pear and raspberry crisp	213	7½	7½
Pimms cocktail jellies	196	3	3
Pineapple and mint cocktail	190	Free	Free
Raspberry marshmallow meringues	202	6½	6½
Speedy summer berry ice	199	3	3
Strawberry and raspberry filo slices	214	3½	3½
Strawberry shortcake sundaes	188	7½	7½
Tiramisu	210	3½	3½
Tropical fruit baskets	215	4½	4½
Tropical fruit rice pudding	208	6	1

Slimming World – the organisation
The complete Food Optimising system and support for your slimming programme is available from Slimming World groups throughout the UK.

If you would like details of the nearest Slimming World class to you telephone our Group Enquiries service on 0844 8978000 between 8am and 8pm from Monday to Thursday, 8am and 6.30pm Fridays.

Slimming World Magazine
As well as running weekly groups, Slimming World also publish *Slimming World Magazine*, the country's largest circulation slimming magazine. It is packed with recipes, menus and success stories. To subscribe, call 0800 1313150 8am and 8pm monday to Friday, 9am and 1am Saturday.

index

acknowledgements

The publisher thanks the photographers and organisations for their kind permission to reproduce the following photographs in this book:

7 Lord Lichfield; 8-9 P. Leggett/SOA; 12-13 Schuster/Robert Harding Picture Library; 14 Brian Limage/The Anthony Blake Photo Library; 15 Tony Robins/The Anthony Blake Photo Library; 16-17 P. Leggett/SOA; 20-21 O. Andrea/Robert Harding Picture Library; 23 Caroline Summers/Scope Beauty; 24 Joff Lee/The Anthony Blake Photo Library; 25 Burkhart/Grazia/Scope Beauty; 26 Lavenstein/Picture Press/SOA; 28-29 P. Leggett/SOA; 30 John Miller/Robert Harding Picture Library; 32-33 P. Leggett/SOA; 36 Gerritt Buntrock/The Anthony Blake Photo Library; 37 Slimming World; 40 Schuster/Robert Harding Picture Library; 41 Joff Lee/The Anthony Blake Photo Library; 44-45 P. Leggett/SOA; 47 Robert Harding Picture Library; 48 Antje Hain/Robert Harding Picture Library; 49 TPH/SOA; 50 Endler/Look/SOA; 46 Scott/100 Cose/Scope Beauty.